6.95

8775

Learning to Nurse

STUDIES IN NURSING SERIES

Already published

Psychiatric Nursing Described
Desmond F.S. Cormack

Ward Sister At Work
Phyllis J. Runciman

Forthcoming title

Postnatal Care — The Midwives' Role
Maureen Laryea

Learning to Nurse
INTEGRATING THEORY AND PRACTICE

Margaret F. Alexander
BSc (Soc Sci) PhD RGN SCM RNT
Senior Tutor/Research Advisor,
Highland College of Nursing and
Midwifery, Raigmore Hospital,
Inverness, UK

Foreword by

Professor A.T. Altschul FRCN
Department of Nursing Studies,
University of Edinburgh,
Edinburgh, UK

CHURCHILL LIVINGSTONE
EDINBURGH LONDON MELBOURNE AND NEW YORK 1983

CHURCHILL LIVINGSTONE
Medical Division of Longman Group Limited

Distributed in the United States of America by
Churchill Livingstone Inc., 1560 Broadway, New York,
N Y 10036, and by associated companies, branches and
representatives throughout the world.

First published 1983

ISBN 0 443 02623 8

British Library Cataloguing in Publication Data
Alexander, Margaret
    Learning to nurse. — (Studies in nursing)
    1. Nursing
    I. Title   II. Series
    610.73   RT41

Library of Congress Cataloging in Publication Data
Alexander, Margaret F.
    Learning to nurse.
    (Studies in nursing series)
    Originally presented as the author's
thesis (doctoral — University of Edinburgh)
    Bibliography: p.
    Includes index.
    1. Nursing — Study and teaching. I. Title.
II. Series. [DNLM: 1. Education, Nursing.
WY 18 A377L]
RT71.A38   1983   610.73'07'11   82–9568

Printed in Singapore by
Selector Printing Co Pte Ltd.

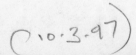

Foreword

Everybody 'knows' that integration of theory and practice in nursing education presents problems. Explanations of why this state of affairs exists abound and so do ideas for remedying it.

Margaret Alexander was, however, not content to accept it as axiomatic that the problem existed, nor was she prepared to treat proferred explanations and solutions as anything other than excuses and clichés. Her analytical mind led her to embark on a rigorous examination of the issue; her longstanding commitment to nursing education caused her not to be satisfied with just investigating it but forced her to do something about it, to carry out action research.

An exploratory survey confirmed that there was a problem. It revealed it in sufficient detail to allow the author to conduct an experiment in teaching which demonstrated that even within the constraints of the existing system of nursing education, nurse teachers can improve their effectiveness.

There is still a dearth of research into nursing education. Margaret Alexander's work makes a very significant contribution to knowledge in a number of ways. First, the results show that students, patients and teachers gain considerable satisfaction when teaching is transferred from the classroom to the bedside, and that this can be achieved in spite of shortage of tutors and within a very short timespan. Second, her research design demonstrated that nursing education is amenable to the same process of measurement and evaluation as are applied to other fields of higher education. Third, she submitted, for the first time in British nursing education, various forms of student assessment to rigorous statistical evaluation, and fourth, she introduces to nursing, developments which have excited higher education since the 1970s. The concept of 'illuminative evaluation' is one which has helped educators elsewhere to escape from the strait-jacket imposed on them by the demands for behavioural objectives. True, nurses were late in discovering Tyler's approach and have only recently learnt to link evaluation with objectives, but this work will help to speed their progress into a more dynamic phase.

Margaret Alexander's work is an in-depth study of an important nursing problem. The account of it, presented in this book, will be of interest to all nurses who recognise how inextricably education, professional development, manpower and standards of care are linked. 1982, when everything in nursing is in the process of change, is a good time to use such an in-depth study as a pivot for one's thinking.

It is my belief that this study is also of interest to educators in all other fields, in particular in all other areas of adult and professional education. One sees references to nursing literature far too rarely in psychological or educational research. I believe it would pay other researchers and practitioners dividends to interest themselves in this study.

Nurse researchers will find this study a veritable goldmine. They would be well advised, when they have read this published version, to delve into the thesis for more detailed information.

To accompany Margaret Alexander through her years of research was like being on an arduous journey. I have learnt more from her than it is possible to acknowledge here. I should like to thank her for introducing me to perspectives on the world of nursing education, the excitement of which I had never before suspected. It is my hope that many readers will also find their nursing perspective newly illuminated.

A.T.A.

Preface

This book, together with the thesis from which it has arisen, is very much a product of the present time in nursing.

Although dealing with events which occurred, and opinions expressed during an educational experiment carried out in six colleges of nursing and midwifery in Scotland, the book constitutes a comment upon certain of the current concerns, and perhaps unrest, in the profession today, as to what it is we are doing and where we are going in nursing, in particular in nursing education.

Fundamental to all that follows are perennial questions, which not only were the springboard for this study, but will hopefully be the springboard for many more in the future. How can we most appropriately prepare recruits to the nursing profession so that standards of patient care will be of the best? How can we achieve an education which is relevant to practice, and which is seen by the student nurse to be something in which he or she is personally involved, an active process of learning which does not *end* with success in the final examinations and registration as a nurse, but continues througout his or her professional life? How can we educate our aspiring nurses so as to help them to develop open minds, a willingness to discuss, adapt and alter both nursing teaching and nursing practice when that is necessary in order to achieve standards of care which will meet the changing needs of individual patients in a changing society?

The book is based upon my thesis, submitted to the University of Edinburgh for the award of the degree of Doctor of Philosophy. Much of the material related to the design of the research, and all of the details of the construction and validation of the multiple choice test designed for the study have been omitted from the book. The recounting of these somewhat prosaic details, while essential in the thesis, has been sacrificed here to permit the inclusion of more of the comments and opinions of those who participated in the research.

Following the presentation, in Part I, of some of the literature related to nurse education and training, to learning — especially learning as relevant to nursing, and to measurement and evaluation in education, Part II gives an outline of the research design and the process of implementation of the experiment. Thereafter, in Part III, the words of the student nurses, the ward staff and the teachers bring alive the evaluation of the experiment, and of the system of nurse education and training in which they work, and give us just a glimpse of some of their thoughts, feelings and values — factors which may be of not a little influence on what they do in their work as nurses. A summary of the findings, and a discussion of some of their possible implications concludes the book.

There are many people whose help, encouragement and understanding are behind this study.

I am indebted to the Scottish Home and Health Department for financial support for this research throughout its course over the three years of my tenure of a Nursing Research Training Fellowship. During that time, Professor Annie T. Altschul, Head of the Department of Nursing Studies, University of Edinburgh, was my main academic supervisor. I am most grateful for her skilled guidance, sustained interest and encouragement, and her unfailing ability to see the wood in spite of the trees. I wish also to record my thanks for the supervision of Dr A.E.G. Pilliner, then Director, Godfrey Thomson Unit for Academic Assessment, University of Edinburgh, who gave kindly and expert assistance in the first year, and to Dr M. Hutchings, then Research Officer, General Nursing Council (Scotland), who took up this task in the third year of the study. My base, throughout, was the Nursing Research Unit, University of Edinburgh, and the support of the Director, Dr Lisbeth Hockey, her staff — in particular Trevor Jones and Dr Hamish Macleod, computer advisers — and of my fellow students was considerable. Miss Elisabeth Hoüe, Director, School of Nursing, Århus Amtssygehus, Århus, Denmark, was a fellow student in the Nursing Research Unit during 1977/78. Her practical help and encouragement during that first year, and especially during the pilot study, was invaluable, and I am grateful for this, and for her continued interest and support throughout the rest of the study.

It was a rare privilege which I deeply appreciated to be able to work with the student nurses, their teachers, the ward staff and the patients, without whose co-operation this research would not have been possible. They responded to this opportunity to give their opinions about nurse education and training, as they knew it, with interest and in quite a number of cases, with enthusiasm. Many took time and thought to give copious comments.

Finally, to my friend, Miss Jem Robertson, Divisional Nursing Officer, Royal Infirmary, Edinburgh, whose support, understanding and whose listening ear were so freely given, and to other friends and to my family who, like Jem, put up with my hermit existence, especially while the thesis and the book were in preparation, I wish to record a most sincere 'thank you'.

So many of the students, in conversation with me after all the stages of the research were over and I was reporting back to them on the results, expressed the hope that their comments would help those coming into nursing in the future. I hope they do.

Inverness 1983   M. F. A.

Contents

List of figures   xiii
List of tables   xiv

PART 1 Learning to nurse *Background and introduction*

1. Introduction to the study   3
2. Nurse education and training: the development and dilemmas of the apprenticeship system   11
3. Theories and concepts of learning applied to nurse education and training   31
4. Measurement and evaluation   52

PART 2 Nursing *An experiment in integration of theory and practice*

5. Context and approach   73
6. Details of the design and the experiment   83
7. The process of implementation   95

PART 3 The research findings

PART 3A *The teaching/learning milieu prior to the experiment*

8. Characteristics of the samples   120
9. Classroom teaching and learning   131
10. Theory and practice   134
11. Ward teaching and learning   140

PART 3B *Evaluation of the experiment*

12. Active experiential learning in nursing: the experiment evaluated in the opinions of the participants   158
13. The experience of the control group students and their teachers   180
14. Results of the tests and essays   184
15. Student nurse study patterns   191
16. Postscript   197

Contd

PART 4 Summary and discussion *Whither nursing?*

   17. Summary and conclusions 203
   18. Discussion and implications: Some answers . . . . but
       more questions? 214

References 226

Further reading 235

Appendix A 238

Appendix B 240

Index 253

List of figures

1. The 'normal distribution'   56
2. A continuum of proficiency   56
3. Distribution 'before and after effective instruction'   57
4. The setting for the research   74
5. The stages of the research   80
6. Pre-test/Post-test control group design   84
7. The design of the experiment   84
8. Essential difference between control and experimental groups   87
9. Typical block day/week   92
10. Control group day/week during experiment   93
11. Experimental group day/week during experiment   93
12. Timespan of main study and date of experiment in each of the five
    colleges of nursing   111
13. College: synopsis of implementation, progress and conclusion of
    experiment   112
14. College: position of experiment in students' training programme   112
15. College: position of experiment in Block programme   113
16. College: control and experimental group experience of course content   113
17. College: teaching methods used for nursing content. Control and
    experimental groups   114
18. Pre-experiment: ward trained staff. Cumulative percentages of numbers
    of trained staff and length of time in present grade   121
19. Pre-experiment: teachers. Cumulative percentage — registered nurse
    teacher — length of time in present grade   124
20. Pre-experiment: teachers. Cumulative percentage — registered nurse
    teacher — length of time as ward sister/charge nurse   125
21. Pre-experiment: teachers. Cumulative percentage — registered clinical
    teacher — length of time in present grade   126
22. Pre-experiment: teachers. Cumulative percentage — registered clinical
    teacher — length of time as ward sister/charge nurse   127
23. Pre-experiment: students. Preference profile — methods of
    teaching/learning   132
24. Pre-experiment: students. Weighted score contribution to ward
    supervision/practical demostration by listed staff grades   144
25. Pre-experiment: students. Weighted score contribution to ward tutorials
    by listed staff grades   146
26. Organised opportunities for study as a proportion of all class periods   193

List of tables

1. Use of wards during experiment   114
2. Movement of students through wards   114
3. Movement of teachers through wards with student pairs   115
4. Pre-experiment: students. Composition of student sample by college   120
5. Pre-experiment: ward trained staff. Distribution of sample by staff grade and hospital   121
6. Pre-experiment: teachers. Distribution of grades throughout colleges   123
7. Pre-experiment: ward trained staff. Frequency of meetings with education staff   128
8. Pre-experiment: students. Recalled examples of practice which differed from what was taught   134
9. Pre-experiment: students. Frequency of supervision/practical demonstration received   142
10. Pre-experiment: students. Frequency of tutorials received   145
11. Pre-experiment: ward trained staff. Frequency of teaching in own ward   147
12. Pre-experiment: teachers. Responsibility for ward teaching   150
13. Pre-experiment: ward trained staff. Responsibility for ward teaching   150
14. Post-experiment: students. Composition of experimental group   158
15. Post-experiment: ward trained staff. Distribution of sample by staff grade and hospital   159
16. Post-experiment: students. Achievement of objectives of experimental method   173
17. Post-experiment: ward trained staff and teachers. Achievement of objectives of experimental method   175
18. Number of students who completed diaries by college and number of days represented in the diaries   191
19. Available classroom periods officially allocated to study   192

PART 1

Learning to nurse
Background and introduction

1

Introduction to the study

How can the integration of theory and practice in nursing be facilitated? To seek an answer to this question was the *raison d'être* for the research upon which this book is based.

There is evidence in abundance, in nursing literature, and in current debate and discussion among nurses, to indicate that integration of theory and practice is a cause of concern in nurse education and training. The lack of integration, the gap between theory and practice, is seen, by many, as an important and pressing problem in nursing. That it is not a new problem will become apparent as the next chapter unfolds, but it was the recognition of this problem by the author, while she was a nurse teacher, which led to her decision to carry out the research. The general aim of the study was to facilitate the integration of theory and practice in nursing. The specific aim was to plan, construct, implement and evaluate an experiment in nurse education. That experiment was the creation of a situation in which student nurses* were given the opportunity to carry out supervised nursing care of patients whose illnesses related directly to the theoretical course of teaching they (the student nurses) were currently receiving. The experiment thus created conditions, as close to the optimal as was possible, to foster an appreciation of positive connections, to forge links between what was taught and what was practised in nursing, to stimulate integration of theory and practice.

Integration, the putting together of relevant parts to make a coherent and meaningful whole, is ultimately an individual matter. The formal organisation of nurse education and training, the introduction of modular programmes, hospital/college of nursing links, certain teaching methods are all aids to integration, but the actual achievement of integration of theory and practice in nursing is seen here as an active, ongoing process, a part of the whole process of

---

* Student nurses have been referred to throughout as 'she'.

learning, and as such, if and when it does occur, is, in essence, an achievement of the individual learner.

Theory and practice defined

The General Nursing Council (Scotland), in their introduction to 'Syllabuses for Nursing' (1973) state:

> The syllabuses set out in general terms the subjects which have to be studied . . . Subjects must be studied both from textbooks and by lectures, but of equal importance is what is learned by working in the hospital and in the community.

In effect, this statement embodies what is meant in this study by 'theory' and 'practice'. Theory is the subject matter of nursing as it is taught in the classroom or college of nursing. It is the material of the formal, or overt curriculum. Practice is what is done when the nurse is engaged in giving nursing care in the wards. It embodies much of what in present day parlance is termed the 'hidden curriculum' (Whitty & Young, 1976), the curriculum which, in nursing, is a potent force in transmitting the values, the beliefs about 'the way nursing is'. There can be no absolute dividing line between theory and practice in nursing, in that, while practising her occupation of nursing, the student will at times be the recipient of *ad hoc* instruction or demonstration in some of the facts or methods of nursing. Although of relevance to this research, such *ad hoc* instruction is not the focus or the prime concern. That concern is with integration of the subject matter of nursing as it is taught in the college with the practice of nursing as it is done in the wards.

THE RESEARCH IN CONTEXT

Nurse education and training in Scotland, as in the United Kingdom, is predominantly based on the apprenticeship model. Since 1976 in Scotland, the formal instruction of the student nurse has taken place in colleges of nursing and midwifery which came into being as a result of the gradual amalgamation of several of the existing hospital schools of nursing and schools of midwifery. Within these newly formed colleges a number of different training programmes were in force leading, for student nurses, to qualification on one or more of the four Registers maintained by the General Nursing Council, i.e. the General, Mental, Sick Children's or Mental Subnormality Registers; for pupil nurses to Enrolment; and for pupil midwives to qualification as a midwife. A few of these colleges brought staff and students together under one roof, but others were a 'college' in name only. Although there was one person in administrative charge, the Director of Nurse Education, the component parts of some of the colleges were in buildings widely separated from each other geographically. In these cases, staff and students from the different parts of the college might never, or only very occasionally meet. For many colleges, the areas where their students gained their practical experience were quite widespread — even perhaps in different towns.

The training programme with which this study was particularly concerned was that which most student nurses experienced in preparing for registration on the general part of the Register. It was the Phase I programme of Comprehensive Training of the General Nursing Council for Scotland. In this programme, the student spent a minimum of 24 weeks in Study Blocks, 8 of which had to be completed within the first 16 weeks of training, and it was recommended that the remainder be completed by 18 months of training. While on secondment to psychiatric, obstetric, paediatric and community nursing, which secondment was an integral part of the programme, a further minimum of 16 days, in Block, study days, or equivalent periods of study was mandatory. This theoretical component was contained within the statutory 144 week training which had to be satisfactorily completed prior to Registration.

The Phase I programme above described is currently in the process of being phased out, to be superseded by a modular programme, in which it is intended that periods of practical (clinical) experience should be immediately preceded by periods of relevant instruction in the college of nursing (General Nursing Council (Scotland), 1978). This closer association of theory and practice, while it is an essential prerequisite, and has considerable potential for the improving of integration of the two, will not of itself deal with many of the fundamental issues. This is stressed, lest the reader consider that, in juxtaposing theory and practice in the formal organisation of a programme, the problem is solved, or that the research described herein is no longer relevant. As will be seen in the following pages, one important first step has been taken, which may well deal with the first two problems described below, but much still remains to be done.

THE PROBLEM — IN OBJECTIVE AND SUBJECTIVE PERSPECTIVE

(1) Clearly, within the system of education and training prevailing during this research (1978–80), it was quite impossible for every

student nurse to leave Block and proceed to directly relevant clinical experience. In a system where students were employees, apprentices, and as such an essential part of the work force on a ward, it was necessary that they be distributed as evenly as possible over all the wards and departments. This meant inevitably that some would go to wards for which they felt they were not specifically prepared. Although it was clear to many of their teachers that it was not possible to provide them with all the knowledge they would ever require, this was not so clear to these young students. This problem of allocation, essentially one of the formal organisation of the programme for each individual student/apprentice, was aggravated by a further factor.

(2) In the majority of colleges of nursing, the organisation of the nurse education was 'syllabus bound . . . subjects given in Block were organised with little thought for what clinical experience the learner may have had, or may be about to have' (Bendall, 1977). There were a few colleges, both in Scotland and in England and Wales where experimental modular schemes of training existed, with the express aim of linking theory with the practical experience which was to follow, but these were the exceptions. For most student nurses, and for their teachers, the arrangement of the teaching followed the organisation of the subject matter of the syllabus, i.e. it was divided into the various body systems and the diseases related thereto.

(3) The allocation of students to particularly labelled clinical areas such as 'medical wards' and 'surgical wards' did not constitute any precise guide as to the experience thus made available to the student. Roper (1976) pointed to inconsistencies in the labelling of wards when compared with the diagnoses of some of the patients within these wards. In her report of a survey of clinical nursing experience available in wards to which students were allocated, she stated:

> The implication for nurse education would seem to be that since there were innumerable learning and teaching opportunities in most clinical areas over and above that which could be expected from the labels, use of such labels as surgical ward and surgical nursing is misleading. (p. 72)

(4) Quite apart from the availability of experience within the wards, a majority of student nurses were unable to learn from the myriad opportunities for learning present in their daily work with patients. Much of the evidence for this statement came from the work experience of the researcher, and from discussions with col-

leagues, some of whom were clinical teachers. The following comment is from a student nurse, who said, of bed-bathing a 56-year-old man, who was cachectic and in the terminal stages of illness caused by gastric carcinoma: 'he was too ill to know who was bedbathing him — I learnt nothing'.

(5) The majority of the trained teachers in nursing were never, or at best only very rarely present in the wards where the nursing was carried out. They were thus never seen to be practising nursing, nor did they teach nursing by doing nursing. Henderson (1966) speaking of her own training days, many years earlier than the date of her book *The Nature of Nursing*, stated:

I seldom, if ever, saw graduate nurses practise nursing — never my teachers. Their teaching was in the classroom. (p. 7)

The situation is little different today. The registered nurse teacher remains, for the most part, cloistered within the college walls. Her colleague, the clinical teacher, attempts to create a bridge between what is taught and what is practised, between the theoretician in the college and the practitioner in the ward — an uneasy position, but one which was created in the 1950s specifically to respond to the needs of the student nurses for teaching while they were working in the wards. But the clinical teachers are too few, many do not remain long in post but move on to take the further qualification necessary to become a registered nurse teacher, and many who wish to remain as clinical teachers are required to spend time teaching in the classroom of the college of nursing — time which must be subtracted from their time in the wards.

(6) As the clinical teacher was drawn into the college of nursing, the subject which she was most often asked to teach was that of 'nursing'. Status for the registered nurse teacher became linked to the teaching of such subjects as human biology, microbiology, and other nursing-related subjects, but not to the teaching of nursing.

(7) Students returning to Block from ward experience frequently complained that what was taught in the college was not done in the wards of the hospital. The same students often became restless at what they saw as the restrictions of remaining in the classroom, when what they wanted was to be back on the wards, yet when they were working on the wards, there was so little time to step back from their responsibilities for giving patient care, and read or ask questions, or really think through what they had been doing.

(8) For the teacher who did go to the wards, to plan and organise learning experiences specifically to encourage the student to integrate her classroom teaching with her ward practice of nursing was

fraught with problems and oft-times doomed to failure, and stressful for all concerned.

Conflict of interests was inevitable, as to teach, whether it be a skill or knowledge, took time, and staffing and pressure of work did not always make that time available.

These then were but some of the factors which are considered to contribute to the problems of integrating theory and practice in nursing, and which led to the research and the experiment described in this book. However:

> the very choice of any research project . . . inevitably presumes an act of judgment in which personal values and personal history play their own — perhaps deep-hidden role. The true science lies in recognising this, not in avoiding the terrain where involvement is most perceptible. (Jackson & Marsden, 1969, p. 17.)

ETHICAL CONSIDERATIONS

There were a number of important ethical issues implicit in this study, involving as it did an educational experiment.

There were obligations to the student.[1] Part of the theoretical component of her training was manipulated and, although her consent to the experiment was requested, the nature of the experiment dictated that it was not possible to inform her fully beforehand of all that was involved. In discussions and negotiations with the college staff, however, the experimental method of teaching/learning could be defended by reference to established theories of learning.

There were obligations to the teachers.[2] For them, involvement meant disruption to their normal working schedule, but also responsibility for the teaching. For some, those who taught the experimental group, this meant teaching in the wards and supervising patient care, with the concomitant responsibilities.

There were obligations to the ward staff. The experimental teaching method set out to use the ward and its facilities primarily for the education of the student nurse, thus involving and requiring co-operation from the large group of trained nurses whose first priority is the care of the patient, and only after that, the education of the learner.

There were considerable obligations to the patient, not least because for some it was not possible, or was deemed unwise, to ask for their consent to participate in the research. There were others who were fully informed and consenting recipients of care. Steps were taken to ensure confidentiality for all patients involved. Students, for example, were asked to be particularly careful about any notes they made, and to use no identifying features which could be traced back to any patient, and the researcher too was careful to ensure that nowhere in the research report was any particular patient identified.

ASSUMPTIONS OF THE STUDY

A number of assumptions underlie this research. These are:

(1) extraneous measures, such as the juxtaposition of theory and practice in the curriculum, the presence of nurse teachers on the wards with supernumerary students, the use of more active rather than passive methods of teaching, will facilitate what is essentially an internal process in the learner, i.e. the process of integration of theory and practice in nursing;

(2) an apprenticeship system of nurse education and training is the preferred method of preparing the greatest number of those who are, or can be, recruited to a labour-intensive service such as nursing is, and no doubt will remain for some considerable time in our society;

(3) the apprenticeship system within this country is a system which is sufficiently flexible to accommodate innovation and change— both large and small scale;

(4) the introduction to the wards of supernumerary, teacher-supervised students whose nursing work is primarily dictated by their needs as students and not primarily by the needs of the ward is not detrimental to the needs of the patients;

(5) problems of perceived lack of integration of theory and practice in nursing are more likely to be a function of the methods of teaching and learning, than of the formal organisation of the training programme. From this premise it follows that ways of facilitating integration should be sought, and can be found, within the current system, rather than by rejecting the entire system; and

(6) the experimental method of teaching/learning would result in a more relevant and more realistic preparation for the daily work of nursing than is achieved by the present predominantly college-based methods.

LIMITATIONS OF THE STUDY

In research, as in life, limitations can be viewed in two ways. The more usual view is of limitations as restrictions — restrictions to interpretation of findings, to generalisation of results. The recognition of such limitations and the creation of a methodology which went some way towards dealing with them, were essential components of the design of this research.

The alternative view of limitation as a challenge also pervades this study. There is the challenge of experiment in such a value-laden area as education; there is the challenge inherent in the attempt to measure learning. Whereas it is relatively straightforward to measure before and after knowledge of a subject, and this was done in this study, it is problematic if not impossible to measure accurately ways of thinking and feeling, opinions and attitudes, yet it is the view of learning as an individual process involving both the cognitive and affective domains which is at the core of this research. The brevity of the experiment in each college, and thus of the individual participants' exposure to the altered teaching method and way of learning would militate against any change in ways of thinking or opinions. Indeed if such changes were, in some cases, initiated, they would prove elusive to identify, more especially as it was not within the scope of the present study to observe behaviour of any of the participants after the experiment took place.

Education and values are inextricably mixed, such is the mix which provides the restriction and the challenge to the research reported in the following chapters.

NOTES

1. The 'students' in this study are student nurses in the education and training programme leading to the qualification of Registered General Nurse (RGN) in Scotland.

2. In Scotland, there are two grades of nurse teacher, therefore where the term 'teacher' appears in the text, this is intended to include both grades, i.e. the registered nurse teacher and the registered clinical teacher. In order to differentiate between the two, where it is the former grade only that is referred to, the term 'tutor' is used, and if the latter only, then the term 'clinical teacher' is used.

2

Nurse education and training: the development and dilemmas of the apprenticeship system

INTRODUCTION

Learning to nurse, for the majority of aspiring nurses in this country takes place, almost entirely, in two separate institutions — colleges of nursing and midwifery, and hospitals. In the former, approximately one-sixth of a basic three year training programme is spent in formal instruction about nursing and related subjects, and in the latter, the remaining five-sixths is spent in working, and thereby gaining practical experience of nursing. Student nurses are employees of the National Health Service, thus the term 'student nurse' is considered by some to be something of a misnomer. However, nurse education and training in Scotland, as in the United Kingdom, is predominantly based upon the apprenticeship model. It is within that model that many of the difficulties related to integration of theory and practice are rooted, yet it is within the same model that the potentials for integration are strong.

EARLY DAYS

The advent of organised nurse training in the United Kingdom 120 years ago was accompanied by opposition and argument. Miss Nightingale had insisted that nurses 'were to have a course of class instruction and practical training in hospital' (Jamieson & Sewall, 1954, p. 337) and the doctors of the time, sensing in these revolutionary proposals a criticism of their own arrangements for the nursing care of their patients countered with the statement that 'nurses were in the position of housemaids and needed only the simplest instruction' (Baly, 1973). Swords were drawn and many would say are still unsheathed, although nowadays the protagonists and antagonists of the various arguments and proposals are to be found much more within the ranks of nursing, and the battle is not over whether any education is necessary, but over what is a relevant education and training for nursing, and of where, when and by whom it should be provided.

11

The origins of the system of nurse education and training which we in this country know today, can therefore be accurately traced to the late 19th century and the ideas and vision of Florence Nightingale. Although at that time the extent of nurse education was minimal by the standards of today, the principle was established and 'in Miss Nightingale's opinion both education and service were integral and equally important aspects of the probationer's training' (SHHD, 1963, p.1). Professor Scott Wright in the Report she compiled for the Scottish Home and Health Department on the Experimental Nurse Training at Glasgow Royal Infirmary, wrote of Florence Nightingale, that in appreciating the need for theoretical as well as practical experience, she saw the significance of one of the main problems affecting basic nurse education today. Scott Wright went on to outline the progress of nurse education and to note the effect upon it of changes in society and in medicine. She cited the development of anaesthetics, and of aseptic surgical techniques as advances which led to demands for many more nurses, which in turn led to a lengthening of the then two year course of training. This change was made under the pretext of giving greater experience, but the labour of young women was very cheap in those days and their services were exploited in a training which had been extended to three years. Brown, writing of this period in 1948, commented: 'if practice made perfect then much could be expected' (p. 49). This emphasis on the practical or apprenticeship aspects of nursing training, and the resulting impoverishment of the educational component, continued until the outbreak of the First World War. Nursing, so much a part of the fabric of society, was caught up in the enormous social convulsion which occurred during and as a result of that devastating war, and its aftermath. The demand had again been for more and more nurses, and for skilled nurses, because further advances in medicine had made it possible to attempt more for the patients. There were insufficient trained and competent nurses to cope with the numbers of sick and injured, but nursing was beginning to reacquire status — to become fashionable again. There was an influx of untrained, or partially trained ladies, anxious to serve their country at a time of such need. Nursing emerged from that war, a profession, but every bit as turbulent and divided amongst its members as the rest of the society of which it was a part.

THE INFLUENTIAL MIDDLE YEARS

In 1919, just after the war, and in an atmosphere of some acrimony, the General Nursing Councils were created. These were statutory bodies, formed to exercise control over the standards in nursing and with the following duties:

1. To compile a syllabus of instruction
2. To compile a syllabus of subjects for examination
3. To compile a register of qualified nurses
   (Baly, 1973, pp. 140–1)

However, it was not from the statutory bodies that the challenge came, in that immediate post-war era. The first post-1919 recommendations for nursing were from the other side of the Atlantic, to which the Nightingale system of nurse education had been exported, in unexpurgated form, some fifty years previously. From the United States of America, the Goldmark Report, dated 1923, recommended a reduction of the three year basic course, by approximately one-quarter, to be achieved by the removal of unnecessary repetition and non-teaching time on the wards. It also broached the idea of college or university-based education for some nurses. This Report preceded the earliest post-First World War evidence in Britain that all was not well with nursing, but in the first Report to be published in this country, that of the Lancet Commission in 1932, there was a rejection of any possibility of a shorter training because it would be detrimental to the hospitals who required the 'probationers' to give service. The Commission did, however, suggest that ward sisters be relieved of some of their duties to enable them to spend more time teaching nurses, but they also stated unequivocally that 'nursing is essentially a craft' (Lancet Commission, 1932, p. 162). Seventy years on, as this Report was, there was almost no sign of Miss Nightingale's plan for a systematic and thorough education for nurses. Although the Lancet Report, of itself, did little to improve the education of the nurse, it became, indirectly, of key importance in nursing because of the considerable reaction and public and professional debate which it stimulated. Many were apparently very dissatisfied with nursing at that time, but then it might have been said that disappointment with developments in nursing was part and parcel of the general disillusionment and disappointment which permeated all of British society in those post-1918 decades. However, for nursing, the decade of the Thirties produced two particularly interesting publications — interesting because of the comprehensive comment they provided upon the contemporary nursing scene and remarkable because, had their publication dates been concealed from a 1980 reviewer, it seems very likely that the concluding summary might have read: 'these books provide a comprehensive comment upon the contemporary nursing scene'.

The books were written by a British doctor and a British nurse, who had herself, some eight years before the publication of her book, given evidence to the Lancet Commission. Dr Balme, writing in 1937, must have been a courageous medical man to write as he did so convincingly, of the necessity to improve the education of nurses. He commented upon the lack of integration of theory with practice, upon the overriding claims of service before education, of the very inadequate provision of bedside teaching, of a crowded syllabus which ignored the social sciences and put a major emphasis on tasks, and of the need for the tutor of nurses to teach her students on the wards, to superintend their work there and to link the symptoms exhibited by the patient with the special nursing application — the nurse should learn why, not just how. He compared nursing preparation to its detriment, with that for physicians, engineers and architects, where a wise combination of practical work and expert instruction gave, in his opinion, better results:

> As a system of education, it (nursing) is almost doomed to failure from the outset, owing to the intense preoccupation of those from whom the young nurse should be receiving the bulk of her instruction. (p. 15)

He was here referring to the ward sister who was so busy that her inexperienced helpers received 'short shrift'. It was not so, he said, for the aspiring doctor.

For the medical student, every effort was made to make him understand why things were being done, but this was a privilege seldom accorded the student nurse. Balme did not know of a single hospital in which regular bedside instruction was given to the nurses, concerning the illnesses and the special nursing methods applicable to each:

> It is only by a happy accident that a lecture will have a direct bearing upon some particular case which a nurse is attending at the moment. (p. 17)

The only anachronism in Dr Balme's text is the use of the term case, or illness, rather than the term patient, and yet he wrote, almost half a century ago, that the nurse soon discovers it is far more important that she learn about people rather than things:

> to understand how to handle human beings (rather) than surgical instruments, but what chance has she of studying psychology in such a crowded syllabus, and what of the social sciences? (p. 20)

He made many recommendations, seeing the need for college or university-type education, perhaps even for grants in the effort to create separation of education from the responsibility for giving service, for more tutors, for faith, finance and a farsighted philanthropist to accomplish the major improvements, but he stressed that much could be done while awaiting radical change:

> It is what is seen on the wards which sticks, and it is a great pity the instruction of nurses is not at present based upon that fact. (p. 54)

Miss Carter, two years later, was preoccupied with many of the problems Dr Balme had mentioned. She too stressed teaching at the bedside and regretted that the Nightingale idea of clinical instruction as 'the bedrock of nurse training' (Carter, 1939 p. 101) had been overlaid by pressure of ward duties, and that:

> the sister tutor, with her time fully occupied by the exigencies of the syllabus, has ... too often been separated from the wards, and in consequence clinical teaching has suffered and with it the bedside care of patients. (p. 111)

She anticipated the present-day Block system in recommending that:

> alternation of work in the wards with periods of study and practice in the school would probably be necessary, but there should never be a complete divorce between theory and practice. (p. 165) The wards would never be shut to her (the student nurse) even while she was taking a course of lectures. (p. 166)

Miss Carter would seem to be a key figure, whose own vision linked the aspirations and ideals of Florence Nightingale with those of present-day nurses and nurse educationists. There was striking parallels between 1860 and today in four matters of which she wrote. These were:

(1) the necessity to precede reforms by careful survey and documentation of the needs of the country for nursing, both preventive and curative;

(2) of the importance to nursing of experiment and research:

> 'there is urgent need now, as there was in 1860, for experiment and research into new methods of nurse training.' (p. 130)

(3) her opinion that education for nursing must be such as to de-

velop reason, the power of association, the faculty of self-expression, and that students should learn principles which they could then apply throughout their training:

'the student nurse has yet to be taught responsibility for her own mind.' (p. 168)

(4) and in this she pre-empts some of the findings of this particular study:

'a reform which would be very attractive to nurses . . . would be the allotting of patients rather than duties to the nurse.' (p. 148)

Such were the issues of the Thirties in nursing — such *are* the issues, almost every one of the important issues, at the threshold to the Eighties in nursing.

TURBULENT FORTIES, FIFTIES AND SIXTIES

Several major landmarks mark the intervening years in nursing, and throughout, in the mass of paper and words, can be distinguished the thread of concern as to what was the most appropriate preparation for the work of nursing. The Horder Committee, reporting in 1943, in the midst of the Second World War, recommended a separation between training and the obligations to provide service for hospital patients, in order that the educational needs of the nurses could take priority and dictate the hospital experience, rather than the reverse, but the Committee emphasised, in heavy type, that they saw 'nothing incompatible between apprenticeship and studentship' (Edwards, 1962 p. 9).

The twin problems of balance between education and service, between theory and practice, were to come under scrutiny from a slightly different angle. The perspective of the Fifties was that of job analysis, and the work which nurses did was observed meticulously. The resulting report — the Nuffield Report on the Work of Nurses in Hospital Wards — shocked the nursing world, and that of the interested public, by it findings. Student nurses were said to be students in name only — 'teaching as such was not found to take up more than a negligible amount of ward time' (Nuffield Provincial Hospitals Trust, 1953 p. 121). During a ward sister's nine hour working day, tuition to student nurses was observed to occupy on average five minutes only, thus:

assuming that the bulk of formal tuition is given to student nurses outside the ward, there is still the question of how the practical work is taught and how it is related to the theory learnt elsewhere. (p. 121)

In the search for, and the finding of an answer to that very question, there was created in nursing a new post, and a new, subtle and far-reaching problem. The struggle for a better balance between education and service, between theory and practice, which until this point had focused upon two key figures in the student nurses' world, the ward sister and the sister tutor; and upon the problems of time and teaching preparation for the former and the isolation from the wards of the latter, changed direction. In a sense, defeat was accepted, and the clinical teacher was born. Between the expert practitioner, i.e. the ward sister, and the trained teacher, i.e. the sister tutor, came the third figure, also a nurse, and one who was charged with the responsibility to integrate theory and practice, to help the student nurse make the link between what was taught and the necessary application of that to practice, between what went on in the classroom and what went on in the hospital. While the positive aspects of the clinical teacher role and function were considerable, her existence almost as an emissary between two opposing camps confirmed the existence of these two camps and in many ways would seem to have increased the area of no-man's-land between them, an area occupied somewhat uneasily by the nurse — some time student, some time apprentice, and by the teacher who was also a practitioner and expected to combine the skills required of both roles.

The year 1956, which in Scotland saw the creation of the post of clinical teacher, saw another important development as a direct result of recommendations arising from a study of the Nuffield Job Analysis. This was a pioneering experimental scheme of nurse training conducted in Glasgow Royal Infirmary. The main problem which that experiment sought to solve was one germane to nursing for many years:

> how may the education of the student nurse be improved without upsetting service obligations to the patient. (Scott Wright, 1961 p. 1)

The direct and principal objective of the experiment was the improvement of patient care, and this was to be attained indirectly by making the training more attractive to the nurse both professionally and personally. The experiment was established on three basic principles — the students should be supernumerary, the whole course should provide the opportunity for linking the theory and practice of nursing and the school of nursing should be economically independent of the hospital. There was a complete break with the usual apprenticeship system of training in that patient care was given only in conformity with the needs of the students for practical experience and not in answer to the needs of the hospital. The students were supervised in giving patient care by their tutors and clinical teachers. The experimental course reduced the time taken to train to two years, instead of the usual three years, and was the first example in this country of a broad-based evaluation of results in terms of the original objectives of the experiment. In common with many evaluation studies today, Professor Scott Wright and the Assessment Committee set up to evaluate the experiment found it difficult to measure the subjective objectives, in terms of the contribution made by the experimental nurses to improved patient care, and relatively easy to measure success in tests and Final State Examinations, and effects upon wastage rates. They had been a little disappointed to find that, on the whole, the experimental course students did not perform so adequately as staff nurses, in their third or 'interne' year, as did students who were a product of the conventional form of training. This was attributed to a lack of progressive responsibility and of clinical experience in the experimental course. In their efforts to diminish 'the "evils" of the apprenticeship form of training . . and to educate students *for* service rather than *by* service the curriculum planners have over-emphasised the theoretical at the cost of the practical aspect of the course' (SHHD, 1963 p. 147). However, they demonstrated that it was possible successfully to prepare student nurses for the Final Examinations in two years, given control of their education and the integration of theory with practice, although it should be pointed out that the student nurses in the experimental course did have 'above average ability' as measured by previous examination successes and/or standard intelligence tests. In some part due to the success of the Glasgow experiment, and in part due to the considered inadequacy of the existing pattern of nurse education to meet the needs of society in that time of accelerating rate of change, the Platt Committee was set up by the Royal College of Nursing in 1961 with the very wide remit to consider the whole field of nurse education. Platt's recommendations, made in 1964, were extensive, and in many ways followed on from the results of experiments both in Canadian nursing and in Glasgow. They supported the view that the school of nursing should be independent of the hospital, with an identity separate from the hospital, and that there should be controlled integration of theory and practice in a course of training which took two years, followed by a third year in which the student gained practical experience. They differentiated between the education of the student nurse and that of the pupil nurse, the former to be concerned more with principles and their applications, and made recommendations to raise the standard of entry qualification for students. However, their most talked-of and controversial recommendation, for which, as it transpired, neither the profession nor the country was ready, was that nurses in training should receive an educational grant throughout their first two years of training — the division should be clear. They were to be students and not apprentices. Platt was 'shelved'. Experimental schemes however continued, building upon not only the Glasgow experiment, but also upon some aspects of Platt, notably the '2 plus 1' format of two years of education plus one year of practical experience, but without the independence inherent in a student grant. Also, somewhat surprisingly, almost all of the developments or experiments were carried out with students of above average educational attainment. Why solutions to the problems in nursing education and training should have been sought in experiments not readily translatable into the everyday world of nursing is, in retrospect, a little difficult to understand, but this may have been a function of the fact that this was a fairly early stage of research in nursing.

SEARCHING FOR SYNTHESIS IN THE SEVENTIES

Nursing education and nursing service entered the decade of the Seventies divided, confused, and at odds with each other, rather than as two co-operating and interdependent groups within nursing, and the profession as a whole faced the prospect of yet another official enquiry — this time commissioned by the then Government and with terms of reference which read:

> to review the role of the nurse and midwife in the hospital and the community and the education and training required for that role, so that the best use is made of available manpower to meet present needs and the needs of an integrated health service. (HMSO, 1972 p. 1)

The Briggs Committee, for so it came to be named (after the chairman, Professor Asa Briggs) saw the last phrase of their remit as distinguishing their enquiry from that of previous groups. From this it can be inferred that the needs of the society had become articulated as a need for integration, for putting together the fragmented parts of the Health Service into an integrated structure for health care.

Within this Committee's most comprehensive Report and recommendations published in 1972, the theme of integration is paramount, from what amounted to what might be termed a macro-concept of integration in terms of the National Health Service as a whole, to a micro-concept in terms of details related to nurse education and training. They state:

> Since nurses and midwives constitute the largest group of National Health Service staff, the success of integration policies will depend substantially on their effective education and deployment. (HMSO, 1972 p. 1)

Within a new pattern of education, they clearly indicate their belief in nursing education as a process of continuing learning which should take place in a variety of clinical settings, i.e. hospital and community, and include the care of all age groups. Apart from confirming the necessity for a small number of entrants to nursing to be educated at university, or college of further education level, they recommend a basic course, common to all entrants to nursing in which 'theoretical instruction should be related step by step to the relevant practical instruction' (p. 86). 'Basic skills can be learnt thoroughly, we believe, only in clinical practice' (p. 86). The Briggs Committee saw it as essential to nursing to attract, and appropriately educate, entrants of very different temperament and ability, and thus, for those more able, there was to be a post-certificate course, which in the case of general nursing would lead to Registration and the possibility of further more advanced courses and specialisation.

> We wish to stress that Registration is not the end of the story for the modern nurse and midwife or for the nurse and midwife of the future. The education of nurses and midwives is a continuous process. (p. 93)

The formal organisation of nursing education was recommended to be within a 'modular system in which each module of training involves concurrent theoretical and practical work. After being given theoretical instruction, students go on to wards to practise what they have learned before they learn something else' (p. 68). The proposed modular system, along with the principle of continuing education, presupposed teaching in or close to the clinical situation and to this end they comment upon the preparation and responsibilities of nurse teachers. They recommend:

direct interrelationships under the modular system of learning
between teaching in the colleges of nursing and midwifery and
in the ward and the community. No teacher would be entirely
based in college or in the clinical situation . . . we also wish to
get completely away from what has become the traditional conception of the nurse tutor, a maid of all work required to teach
all subjects in the nursing syllabus. We believe that this conception is inapplicable in present and future circumstances. It
can no longer satisfy the individual concerned nor provide the
right approach to teaching for students. (p. 111)

In pinpointing the generalist role of the nurse teacher, the Briggs
Committee, on the one hand, highlights one of the major difficulties for the nurse teacher in undertaking ward teaching, and on the
other, takes account of the increasing incidence of highly special-
ised nursing required today. The Committee does not consider that
the nurse teacher alone should be responsible for nurse teaching,
but recommends that clinical nurses at ward and community level
should teach both in the clinical situation and in the college.

Briggs' far-reaching recommendations for nursing education
stemmed from the identification of certain fundamental problems,
three of which have direct relevance to this study. These were:

the ambivalent position of the nurse in training both as learner
and worker; determining the balance of theoretical and practical
work in the learning process itself; and the dual role of the
hospital as the provider of nursing care for patients and the
provider of education for nurses. (p. 64)

In expressing these three dichotomies, Briggs brought into focus
once more matters which had bedevilled nurse education since its
inception.

Why are these divisions so resistant to the passage of time and
the changing resources and needs of society? To a great extent, it
must be because they are inherent in the concept of nursing, nursing which means so many different things to different people in
different circumstances. Fundamentally, nursing means caring, yet
caring with sufficient insight so as not to diminish but if possible
enhance the independence and self-respect of the recipient of that
care; nursing means teaching, teaching patients, their relatives and
teaching one's own colleagues; and nursing means organising, organising the appropriate ways and means to achieve the two former
elements of the task which is nursing. It is not the intention in this

book to enter the debate in regard to 'what is nursing' — suffice to state that it is one of the most diverse occupations in our society. There are nurses in acute wards and fast-moving highly technical intensive care areas in hospitals; there are nurses in tranquil hospices for the care of those terminally ill; there are nurses in the sterile, impersonal atmosphere of the operating theatre, and nurses in the very personal atmosphere of the patient's own home. The only common denominator is that nurses work with people, healthy and ill, young and old, in this process of caring and teaching. To do this well, there is consensus that nurses must be educated. Beyond that, there is no consensus.

The dichotomies discussed

Nursing literature abounds with evidence of the three dichotomies, of the gap, nay the gulf between (a) theory and practice, or what is taught and what is practised in nursing, (b) education and service, or the college of nursing and the hospital, and (c) the position of the nurse as a student and as an apprentice.

Research evidence of discrepancies between theory and practice

From 1960 onwards research into nursing began to make an increasing contribution to the literature on the above-mentioned dichotomies. Early preoccupations in nursing research were with reasons for withdrawal from training, or excessive absenteeism, and one of the causative factors was considered to be the discrepancy between what was taught and what was practised. Dalton (1969), in a study of those who had withdrawn from training for the mental subnormality register, reported that over 60% of her respondents found that teaching was generally inconsistent with practice on the wards. In the same year, MacGuire had documented similar complaints by student nurses, and some three years later Birch (1972) associated withdrawal with, among other factors, stress and conflict for the learner arising from differences between classroom and ward practices of which he commented: 'conflict in this area appears to be one of the greatest undermining influences in training' (p. 108). He also felt that 'it was totally unjustifiable to close one's eyes to this complex matter . . . (and suggested that) all teaching of nursing care be done on the wards rather than in the practical room' (p. 169). Hunt, in 1971, found disturbing evidence of potentially dangerous nursing practice in the carrying out of surgical dressings. Not only did practice in a number of cases differ from the theoretical procedure taught in the classroom, but the differences violated aseptic principles. An equally disturbing study, by Jones (1975), ex-

posed differences between teaching and practice in regard to feeding of unconscious patients which resulted, not only in patients
receiving inadequate nutrition, but also in very dangerous technique
in the procedure of administering the feeds. Many have been the
reasons put forward to account for the discrepancies. Roper in 1976
blamed the system to a certain extent: 'The Block system seemed to
have produced increasing disparity between theory and practice'
(p. 2). Abdel-Al (1975) found 'theory and practice unrelated in
terms of administration, time sequence and distribution of content
and sometimes of principles' (p. 545) — a complex matter indeed.
She went on to define the problem more fundamentally as a lack of
representation of the reality of the practical situation in teaching.

The ideal and the reality
There are two aspects to the problem of differences between classroom teaching and ward practice. If the reality is of low standards
of nursing care, and unsatisfactory practice, then it is undesirable
that teaching should reflect that reality, and the solution to the
problem of differences should be sought in the wards and with the
ward staff. In such circumstances, the teacher may be correct and
the ward incorrect. On the other hand, teaching may be unrelated
to ward practice which is perfectly satisfactory and sufficiently
flexible to cope with changing demands and nursing problems. In
these circumstances, the solution should be sought in the college
and with the teachers, and measures instituted to promote more
relevant teaching.

The existence of an ideal and a quite separate reality had been
described in 1973, by Bendall, then Registrar of the General Nursing Council for England and Wales, and a prolific writer and
researcher in nursing education. In a study which was to prove very
influential in nursing, Bendall (1973) produced data which indicated
that, for many nurses, what they wrote in examinations did not predict what they would subsequently do in practice in the wards, i.e.
their recall of theory was at variance with their application of that
theory. This was very disturbing evidence of a widening gap
between theory and practice, the ideal and the reality of nursing.
Bendall did not find that correlation between what was written and
what was practised was aided by relevant theory given at the same
time as practice, but she did claim that 'if the school's teaching is
reasonably in harmony with what goes on in the ward, correlation is
more likely' (Bendall, 1973 p. 127).

Hutchings (1981) contends that Bendall's statistical analysis does
not support the conclusions she makes, although he does not dis-

pute that written examinations are of only limited value in predicting practical performance in nursing.

Could it be that nurse education was becoming an end in itself, building up a body of knowledge unrelated to the actual practice of nursing?

Hughes et al (1973) state, with reference to the preparation of students for the professions of medicine, law, theology and social welfare, that the goals of education and service do not always mesh and that pressures of work may lead to 'bad habits'. Different priorities and different values held by those in education and service have been the subject matter of many other writers. Martin (1973) quotes a student nurse's comment in this respect:

> It is the hospital not the school which is the dominant influence in the student nurse's existence. (p. 114)

Dodd (1974) considered the school and the nurse teacher as almost irrelevant to the student nurse, who valued the ward as the 'real' situation. Harrison et al (1977) in a report describing factors influencing integration of theory and practice in modular schemes of training state:

> a fundamental assumption underlying the idea of integration is that whilst teachers and service staff by necessity have different priorities, they can come together and agree the main educational aims and ways of attaining them. We should not underestimate the ward sister's ability to influence the student's education. She can not only modify the student's behaviour in the ward, but influence her whole attitude to the value of the educational process. (p. 508)

Kramer (1974) in San Francisco, published results of an eight year study into the 'shock' effects upon newly graduated nurses of the discovery of discrepant value systems between school and hospital. In this country, the equivalent would be not the newly registered nurse, but, because of our apprenticeship system of training, the student, fresh from the Introductory Block, who emerges to work on the wards, prepared in the school for an ideal which does not materialise in practice. It is her resulting disillusionment, or 'shock' which has, to some extent, prompted both of the investigations by Birch (1972 and 1978) and which was the stimulus to at least one ongoing study by Gott (1979).

The seclusion of tutors — and of ward sisters
One factor thought by many to be contributory to the existence of

disparate values between education and service is that of the virtual seclusion of the nurse teachers within the college setting, and the fact that the other very important teachers of nurses, the ward sisters, are almost equally secluded within their own setting of the hospital. Few of the latter group are to be found teaching in the college, and, in a situation where teachers are almost completely absent from the scene of real nursing, variations in views on nursing practice such as Lamond found in 1970, in her examination of the process of becoming a nurse, are inevitable.

The General Nursing Council for Scotland, in 1976, reported on evidence they had submitted to the Royal Commission on the National Health Service, and said:

> We do not believe that any teacher of the practical activity of nursing should be so divorced from the practical situation as this group (the Registered Nurse Teacher) is at present. This opinion is shared by student nurses who have stated that their teachers do not come sufficiently often to the wards. (General Nursing Council (Scotland) 1976 p. 21)

Altschul (1978) stated that nursing education was becoming almost irrelevant to patient care, that the teacher of nurses 'away from the ward and unable to obtain any feedback from the students of the effect of her teaching' made no significant input to patient care. Ferguson (1976) queried: 'If nursing is essentially practical, can it properly be taught by people who do not nurse?'.

To return to the realities of practice would not be easy for many nurse teachers. Many are themselves the product of the pre-Block days in nurse training when lectures often were attended in the students' precious off-duty hours and the struggle was to attain a separation between the educational component of training and the practical experience. Many such teachers fear a loss of hard-won 'rights' in a return to teaching in the wards. In addition, the longer a teacher has remained in the school, perfecting her skills as a classroom teacher, the less she has utilised those skills which are paramount in the ward. There are other difficulties entailed in the transfer of some of the teaching/learning experiences from the classroom into the ward. Abdel-Al (1975) found when introducing her 'reality-based' instruction in a school of nursing that tutors did not have time to teach on the ward 'due to other commitments' (p. 255) for example the formal organisation of work in a school of nursing can make it impossible for tutors to have any regular pattern of attending wards. The straitjacket of the syllabus and the timetable can however give a measure of security to the tutor which is absent from the unpredictable though rich variety of learning experiences available in the wards. Houe (1978), following a study of ten nursing schools in this country, considers one major disincentive to teaching in the wards derives from the generalist role of most teachers in colleges of nursing, and she contrasts this with the specialist role of their colleagues who teach in university courses or colleges of higher education. She states:

> While teachers in universities and colleges of higher education teach mainly within their field of interest and skill, and teach in the wards as well as in the classrooms, this is not the common role of the teacher in a hospital-based school. These teachers are not working as specialists but are expected to teach a number of different subjects and these they teach almost entirely in the classrooms; very few have teaching commitments in the wards. (p. 88)

However, coming as she does from another of the EEC countries, Denmark, where there is only one grade of nurse teacher, and where her own particular experience is of teachers who teach nursing in both college and ward, Houe concludes her brief discussion of the gap between theory and practice, education and service in this country, with the simple question: 'why two types of nurse teacher?' (p. 89).

The clinical teacher

Clinical teachers arrived on the scene of nursing education in the mid-fifties, as has been previously mentioned. Robertson (1979) considers they were introduced in an attempt to integrate theory and practice and 'in response to the need for more systematic ward teaching and a shortage of nurse tutors to provide it', and that they indeed make a crucial contribution to integration. Kirkwood (1979), on the other hand, points to the many anomalies current in the role of the clinical teacher and queries whether, although she has served nursing education through a difficult period, this period is not now over and the nurse teacher of the future 'must combine the skills of both roles; that of theoretician and clinician'.

The current situation in nurse education is certainly changed since the 1950s, in particular in regard to the increased numbers of those whose first responsibility is to the learner and her teaching. Ratios of teachers to learners in Scotland have steadily improved to a present figure of 1 : 19, and there are a number of experimental training schemes. In addition the climate of opinion within nursing generally is such that some are beginning to question the continued necessity for the clinical teacher. The General Nursing Council (England and Wales) has agreed to the gradual replacement of the present system of two grades of nurse teacher with a single post of 'teacher of nursing', although their Scottish counterparts remain committed to the continuance of the two grades.

Sequencing of theory and practice

The most recent efforts of the General Nursing Councils in both England and Scotland, in pursuit of their general aim to bring theory and practice, education and service closer together, have been directed towards the promotion of modular schemes of training.

A widely acknowledged fault of the Block system was that periods of theory and of relevant practice had often been widely separated (General Nursing Council (Scotland) 1978 p. 2). In 1971, Bendall had published research which dealt with the sequencing of theory and practice, and the influence of the ordering of these aspects of nurse education upon student learning. She had investigated the policy, practice and opinions in regard to the relationship of theory to practice in a random sample of training schools in England. Tutors, ward sisters and student nurses were strongly in favour of theory before practice (72% to 85% in favour in the three groups), and although a policy in this regard existed in a majority of the schools studied, in actual practice a high proportion of student nurses (95% in second year and 87.5% in third year) had worked in wards prior to having appropriate theoretical preparation. Thus, she concluded, there may be 'considerable discrepancy in many hospitals between what is said to be done and what is done; . . . and students are caught between training and service' (Bendall, 1971 p. 171). It seemed logical to test whether there was any difference in learning between groups of students having a different order of theory and practice and between groups having a different time interval between theory and practice. Bendall's results showed that order was of value in terms of learning efficiency provided the time interval between theory and practice was not more than six months, and where some form of sandwich, i.e. theory, practice, theory, could be devised, learning would be further enhanced. Learning was assessed in this study using objective tests which had been devised and tested for reliability by the researcher.

Already at the time of Bendall's research, experimental modular schemes of training were being planned and implemented both north and south of the Border and in 1972, the Briggs Committee clearly recommended the system. In December 1978, in Scotland, the General Nursing Council, following extensive consultations with both nursing education and nursing service personnel issued new schemes of training which were to apply to all four parts of the Register of Nurses, i.e. General, Mental, Sick Children's and Mental Deficiency. These schemes were wholly committed to the principles of modular instruction, and to the joint responsibility of education and service staff to provide for the education of the learners.

The new scheme requires that periods of clinical experience should be immediately preceded by periods of relevant instruction. The close association of theory and practice should lead to the achievement of a continuous educational programme. Council considers it of the highest importance that the educational nature of the student nurse's clinical experience should be realised, as her employee status is acceptable only on this understanding. (General Nursing Council (Scotland) 1978, p. 4)

Council recommended that both grades of teacher and members of the service staff should be involved in formulating objectives for each clinical period, thus acknowledging the necessity for information about, and understanding of, the concept inherent in the new scheme of education to be shared between the two groups from the beginning. But new schemes, and recommendations, just as reports, are not self-executive.* The close association of theory and practice will not necessarily lead to more realistic teaching, nor to the use of teaching methods which aim to promote integration of theory and practice. Perhaps most importantly of all, the modular schemes do not require that the teacher of nursing in the college should also practise nursing.

Teaching and practice combined
In this regard, a most interesting experiment in nurse education and training, which would appear to be the first of its kind in England and Wales, and in which the work of the clinical teacher and the registered nurse teacher was identical, has been recently reported. The experiment took place within the introductory course in a college of nursing and entailed the greatest amount of the course content being taught by the teachers, not in college, but in the hospital, and on the wards, while supervising the introductory course students. In a comprehensive evaluation of the scheme,

---

* Marginalia on the Draft of the Sanitary Commission on the Health of the Army. F. Nightingale, July 1857. Quoted in Baly (1973)

Taylor stated that although 'the New Style Course has more than trebled the time spent on clinical experience in previous courses, yet no suggestion of any reduction in this area was received' (Taylor, 1979, p. 79). The writer was here commenting on the post-course opinions of the involved teachers. She continued: 'in this study the work of tutors and clinical teachers is seen as identical. Meeting the needs of a student in Introductory Course does not lend itself to a differentiation of duties' (p. 87). This particular scheme of education and training, had several features which were akin to the research experiment which is described in this book, e.g. the identical roles of the two grades of teacher, the intention in the evaluation to obtain the views of all three groups of participants, and not least that the nurse teachers were present and teaching in the wards, helping the students make the link between practice and theory. The success of the above course, i.e. 'Bolton's Introductory Course' (Kelly, 1980) is confirmed by the fact that it is still extant, two and a half years after it commenced, and that it was deemed of advantage by students, ward staff and teachers. A majority of the students felt more confident and better prepared to begin their practical nursing experience after this course; the teachers, though 'tired', valued the method and felt that they were better able to appreciate the ward staff's problems; and the ward staff also approved the scheme and felt they had gained an increased understanding of the role of the teacher.

WHAT OF THE EIGHTIES?

Is it in the type of teaching described above, involving as it does collaboration and communication between teachers, ward staff and students that the best possibilities for improved integration of theory and practice will be found? Such teaching is not dependent upon any one method of formal organisation of the nurse education and training programme, but can operate equally well in the traditional or the modular programmes. What happens within nursing education and training in the 1980s will depend upon the continuing understanding and commitment to the 'new scheme' objectives by all in education and service. Only thus can a climate conducive to learning be attained in both school and ward. The facilitation of integration, which is active learning by the student, will make demands upon the teachers, who must move out of the relative security of the college and into the wards and endeavour to help the student apply theory to practice; it will make demands upon the ward staff who must not only cope with, but encourage the thinking, questioning student; and it will make demands upon the student to become actively involved in the process of learning to think about nursing. Strohmann (1977) pointed to the necessity to shift the emphasis in nursing education from the doing to the thinking aspects of learning.

Fundamentally integration means thinking:

> integration (synthesis) must take place in the head (intellectual processes) of the student. (Halliburton, 1976, p. 53)

Brotherstone (1960) has said:

> There is a general human unwillingess to disturb the quiet sleep of traditional practice. Thinking is often a painful process, and most of us prefer to abstain. (pp. 24–25)

If integration of theory and practice in nursing is inseparable from the process of thinking — perhaps this is why integration has eluded us all in nursing for so long.

3

Theories and concepts of learning applied to nurse education and training

In this chapter, theories and concepts of learning are considered, always in relation to learning to nurse, and to nursing. Inevitably, because teaching and learning are closely linked, the role of the teacher is touched upon at some points.

Learning to nurse is learning to care — learning to care for people; whole people, not 'parts' of people such as a fractured skull, an ampulated limb, a gastric ulcer; but individuals of different appearance, with different ways of behaving, with often vastly different experiences of life as a result of which they have different problems and accomplishments, sadnesses and joys, fears and faiths. Any or all of these aspects of a person's life experience may have some bearing on how they react to whatever event has brought them into the nurse's care. Learning to nurse means learning to cope with unpredictability, because people, sick or well, are unpredictable.

Hockey (1980) in a paper entitled 'Challenges for Nursing' described the challenge for teachers of nurses as the necessity that they educate for care. Within a comprehensive definition she included education for empathy, for respect of the individual, education in the application of theory to practice, in decision making, in manual skills and in 'education for change'. A tall order indeed, and the other side of the coin depicted in the above paragraph, from which it can be deduced that nursing involves activities in the three domains of behaviour described by Bloom (1956), i.e. the cognitive, affective and psychomotor domains. If one accepts the views given above, then learning to nurse is concerned with the gaining of knowledge and the development of intellectual skills and abilities (the cognitive domain), it is concerned with the development of attitudes, values and the ability to adjust adequately in order to cope with different situations (the affective domain), and it is concerned with the development of skilled and dexterous manual techniques (the psychomotor domain).

EDUCATION OR TRAINING?

Is learning to nurse more appropriately described as an education or as a training? Is learning to nurse neither one nor the other, but both? If it is both, should there be emphasis upon one or the other, upon education or upon training? That there exists in the minds of most people a distinction between these two concepts is implied in the manner in which the two words are used in our daily language. We commonly hear of vocational training and general education, or of professional training and liberal arts education. Glaser (1962) considered both education and training were a part of the instructional process, thus concerned with the modification and development of student behaviour, but whereas the training component was concerned to minimise individual differences as for example in teaching students to perform uniform behaviours such as adding, or reading, the educational component was concerned with maximising individual differences, that is accepting and exploiting the fact that some students will add more quickly, read more expressively, as a result of other factors quite extraneous to the training situation. Glaser continued to explain what he considered as the more usual distinction between education and training in terms of 'the specificity of the behavioural end-products'. When an end-product can be precisely specified in particular student performance then instructional procedures can be designed to build in such behaviour, i.e. to train the student. When the end-product behaviours are too complex to specify exactly, or when the behaviour which results in successful accomplishment cannot be known in many instances, then the student is expected to transfer his learning to the performance of the behaviour it was found difficult to analyse. To help him do this, he must be educated.

Viewed in the terms outlined by Glaser there is no doubt that learning to nurse involves problems of both education and training. There are specific behaviours, analogous to those mentioned by Glaser — the student nurse must learn to calculate drug dosages, to accurately complete a fluid balance chart; she must learn about aseptic technique in order to handle forceps, handle a syringe, change an intravenous infusion flask, but the application of these techniques will involve very different behaviour depending upon the people, the patients involved. The application of aseptic technique in the catheterisation of a patient, already anaesthetized and in the near sterile atmosphere of the operating theatre will require quite different behaviour from the successful application of the same technique in catheterizing an elderly lady with severe rheumatoid arthritis in bed in a ward (or in her own home). The latter task requires the student to maximise her creative ability to perform her nursing skills, to apply her knowledge. MacMillan (1980) differentiated education and training in an article which began 'You're not paid to think, just get on with the job.' She equated education with a 'whole person' approach, the student thinking things out for herself, whereas training was essentially task-oriented and did not embrace the 'whole person' concept.

Bendall (1975) writing on the subject of learning in Raybould (1975) appeared to distinguish between education and training in terms of the different teaching methods which were predominantly associated with the learner's status as a student or as an apprentice. Training she equated with learning by doing the job under the supervision of someone already trained (the apprentice) and education with attending lectures, discussions, seminars, whereby knowledge was imparted (the student).

Vickers (1973) states: 'no sharp line divides the education of the individual generally . . . from his preparation for a specific vocation.' He does, however, see dilemma and conflict between the demands, within any educational system, for testable skills and knowledge and for less testable but more fundamental skills and attitudes, i.e. between the overt and the covert curriculum — in that 'the best way to teach the second is not always the quickest way to teach the first.' Again this dilemma would seem so relevant in nursing, in that the best way to teach in order to promote transfer of learning is not always the quickest way to 'cover the content of the syllabus' or indeed to prepare the students for the most easily testable, i.e. knowledge as required to pass the examination for qualification to register as a trained nurse. It is also in nursing relatively easy to test the step by step performance of a skill such as the giving of an injection, in the classroom, and into a 'dummy' or — equally insensitive — into an orange, but problematical to define and test all that is implied in the successful accomplishment of that skill with a patient.

Thus there are three areas of uncertainty for the teacher of nursing: the learning process itself with its possibilities, its limitations and its individual variety; the society, the National Health Service and the requirements of the Syllabus for Nurse Training within which he or she must operate; and the future in nursing — not just nursing as it may be in the next decade, because trainee nurses are all too soon 'fully-fledged', but nursing in the year 2000, which is when many of today's trainees will be the leaders, the decision makers, in nursing. However, although it is important to bear in mind that learning to nurse takes place within the context of all these areas of uncertainty, it is the process of learning which is of central importance in this chapter.

NO SINGLE THEORY

Just as no single theory of learning can account for all learning, so there can be no single theory which can entirely account for all learning in relation to nursing. There is a formidable and growing mass of literature on learning theory, which has become a distinct area within the subject matter of psychology. At the turn of the century, and through into the 1940s two major schools of thought predominated in the psychology of learning. These were the stimulus-response associationists and the cognitive-field theorists (Goodwin & Klausmeier, 1975; Roueche, 1975).

Stimulus-response theory viewed learning primarily as the establishment of bonds between certain stimuli and certain responses. It was concerned with observable elements in the learning process, with behaviour change which could be seen to have occurred in response to a specific stimulus. The emphasis was upon the measurable, upon strictly controlled laboratory conditions, and, although there was an acceptance by leading proponents of this school of the existence of 'internal mental operations' within the mind of the learner, these operations were almost totally ignored. They were unobservable, therefore unknown and unsuited as scientific data (Goodwin & Klausmeier, 1975). Inevitably, from such a perspective, man was viewed in a somewhat passive role, reacting to a determining environment (Bigge, 1971). In contrast, in cognitive-field theory, man was seen as purposive and interacting with his environment. The Gestalt school, as the cognitive-field theorists came to be known because of their stress upon the total situation or 'Gestalt', stressed that the individual's internal cognitive operations were of primary importance in learning, and relegated the mere pairing or associating of a stimulus or response to a secondary position. Although these two schools would appear to be far apart and differing fundamentally in their view of learning, Goodwin & Klausmeier consider the difference to be more one of emphasis. Cronbach (1977) also refers to a difference in emphasis only, in what he terms the 'behaviorist-humanist dialectic'. He considers the two lines of thought complementary — the former analytical and precise, the latter integrative and broad. Of the behaviorist, he states:

Strict behaviorism places exceptional emphasis on what can be seen, and so, on what can be recorded objectively. Reasoning is cautious, and conclusions are limited to observable behavior. The strict behaviorist speaks only about what a person *does*. He avoids reference to the mind, the feelings, or any other inner state. (Cronbach, 1977, p. 19)

Of the humanist:

The humanistic psychologist prefers the very language the behaviorist avoids. His psychology is particularly concerned with inner states, feelings, aspirations, the self. The humanist sees each person as a self-directing, integrated being, evolving in a unique direction as he interprets his experiences. Although the humanist psychologist, like any other, seeks to ground his reasoning in thorough observation, the subject himself is a key observer. (p. 23)

The concepts of the behaviourist — conditioning, both classical and operant, reinforcement, behaviour modification — are as well-known to students of educational psychology as are many of the names. Thorndike described 'trial and error' learning, and the important reinforcing effect of a satisfying response, using a hungry cat in a cage. Pavlov contributed a great deal to knowledge of conditioning with his experiments with salivating dogs. Watson, whom Hills (1979) called the father of the behaviourist movement, drew heavily on Pavlov's work and became convinced that learning was a process of building conditioned reflexes through the substitution of one stimulus for another. Skinner, with his now famous box, variously occupied by a rat, a pigeon or a dog, has long been concerned specifically with the fundamental importance of reinforcement in learning.

Although many of the early experiments of Gestalt psychologists were also conducted with animals, for example Kohler's studies of insightful learning in chimpanzees, members of this school were much more concerned to describe human behaviour in its natural setting. Their key concepts were couched in terms such as understanding, perception, discovery, and insight, and they were interested in the wholeness of the learning experience, within the environment as the learner saw it at the time. This 'life space', as Kurt Lewin termed it, was entirely an individual perception. Two individuals in the same physical environment, say a classroom, could be in very different psychological environments (Munn, 1966), and purposively interacting with their own individually perceived environment in order to pursue their own both short- and long-term goals in what seemed to be the best way to the learner at the time.

It is interesting to see the basic concepts of these two movements persist into the Sixties, although by that time there was a certain merging of the two extreme views into what Cronbach (1977) termed an intermediate position. This, his own position, was the cognitive-developmental style which took account more equally of both objective and subjective factors in learning. Entwistle & Hounsell (1975) place learning theories along a continuum ranging from behaviourist to humanist from tight control, objectivity and measurement, to freedom, subjectivity, exploration. These writers also place methods of teaching or instruction on a similar control/explore dimension and suggest that it may thus be possible to identify some of the theoretical ideas underlying different forms of teaching.

EXTRINSIC MOTIVATION — THE 'POKER-CHIP' MILIEU

Quite clearly at the control end of the continuum in the Sixties were Skinner, and, although not so extreme, Gagné. Skinnerian views are seen in what McKeachie (1975) termed the 'technological revolution in education' — the teaching machine and programmed learning. There can be few schools of nursing which were not swept into the then current craze for this step-by-step learning — the second step contingent upon a correct first step, in fact reinforcement to the extreme. It was a development certainly not unsupported by research — in nursing and elsewhere (Balson, 1969; Guimei, 1977). Many programmes were written by nurses for nurses. Isaacs & Hull (1975), working together in Luton School of Nursing, were particularly prolific writers of programmes, though not all of their work reached publication and therefore general circulation. Although in working through a programme, the learner was actively involved, the main controlling factor was external, within the programme and based upon knowledge of results. But teaching machines have all but disappeared — their failure due, according to McKeachie, to the fact that their proponents did not take seriously enough the research literature on subjective factors such as motivation in learning. In addition research evidence was beginning to sow seeds of doubt about the place of knowledge of results in learning. Sturges (1972) and Kulhavy & Anderson (1972) showed that knowledge of results made little difference and might in some circumstances even be detrimental to learning. A further potent influence on the demise of the pre-eminence of externally controlling factors in learning was the writings of Abraham Maslow.

Maslow believed that 'human nature has been sold short by the dominant psychological theories' (1968, p. 687), with their emphasis on extrinsic learning and what he felt was an inevitable result — the 'poker-chip milieu' (Maslow, 1975, p. 160) of the university where students responded to grades and examinations as chimps to poker chips.

INTRINSIC MOTIVATION AND INDIVIDUAL DIFFERENCE

Writing in 1970, Maslow set out a comprehensive theory of motivation, to explain the 'why' of human behaviour. He posited seven levels of need as directing all human behaviour: physiological, safety, love and belonging, esteem, self-actualization, needs to know and understand, and aesthetic needs. These needs were hierarchical, in the sense that normally, lower order needs, which he referred to as deficit needs, would be satisfied before higher order or growth needs could be met. His is a dynamic concept, however, in that no individual was permanently at one level in all circumstances, but his view of education was of helping a person grow towards realising his full potential. Maslow is perhaps best known for this emphasis on self-actualization, on being or becoming the person we potentially can be, and thus for his emphasis on the importance of the intrinsic learning experience, which is not only highly personal, but conjoins the emotional and the cognitive. Maslow wrote, only two weeks before his death in 1974, 'the thrust of what we are learning in humanistic psychology is the extent of individual differences within the species' (Maslow, 1974, p. 151). The implications for education generally, and nursing education in particular, lay in the acceptance of all the individual differences among students, and the vital importance of helping each student to gain a sense of accomplishment, to encourage creativity and discourage regimentation, to help the student towards meeting his growth needs. Maslow's view of the teacher was therefore not of one who is a shaper of persons, but one who helps a person discover what is already within him, a role which he acknowledges is very difficult and not within the capabilities of all — but even in this he suggests acceptance of individual differences within teachers:

in any group of teachers there will be some who will be comfortable with a Summerhill* approach and some who will not
...I see no reason for not having within conventional school
systems the experimental schools. (Maslow, 1974, p. 165)

His philosophy, in regard to meeting the needs of self-esteem and
self-actualisation, takes on another dimension when applied to
nursing, where the interaction is not only the teacher/student dialogue but also the nurse/patient dialogue. Any method of teaching
and learning nursing which takes place at the bedside has the
potential to provide a sense of accomplishment and thus meet
growth needs not just for teacher and student, but also for the
patient receiving care. In such a situation, the patient, often someone
temporarily deprived of normal opportunities for self-actualization,
for self-esteem, is in many instances enabled to meet his needs in
these respects by teaching the student, indeed both student and
patient may meet the higher order need — 'to know and understand'
more about health and disease. Conversely, the issues of human
dignity and self-respect, so integral to good nursing care, are likely
to evade all but the most perceptive of students if nursing is taught
primarily in a practical room in a controlled but unrealistic situation — 'you simply do not ask questions about ultimate human
values if you are working in a . . . lab' (Maslow, 1968 p. 686).

EXPERIENTIAL LEARNING

The place of the emotions and the personal involvement of the student in the process of learning, which Maslow, and a contemporary
humanistic psychologist Carl Rogers, have stressed, are, in the
opinion of the researcher, particularly apposite to the process of
learning to nurse. Rogers' *cri de coeur* was for freedom to learn, that
the student should be allowed to develop his/her own ideas and to
participate responsibly in the learning process. Rogers divided
learning into two general types, along a continuum of meaning. At
one end he placed the learning of nonsense syllables and contended
that much in the curriculum is equally meaningless for many
students today:

Such learning involves the mind only. It is learning which
takes place 'from the neck up'. It does not involve feelings or

---

* Summerhill Academy was a very progressive school in East Anglia, England,
  founded upon principles and beliefs about education similar to those of Maslow.

personal meanings; it has no relevance for the whole person. (Rogers, 1969, p. 4)

It is salutary to reflect whether Bendall's (1973) evidence of recall of nursing procedures which bore no relationship to the actual application of such nursing procedures in the wards might not be an indication that much of the formal curriculum of nursing as taught in the colleges of nursing is learning from the neck up and as such rather meaningless to many of the students. She stated:

It can be postulated that what was, in this project, recalled had been learned by rote; and what was applied had been learned by discovery. (p. 134)

The contrast, at the opposite pole of the continuum of meaning which Rogers describes, is 'significant, meaningful, experiential learning'. The elements of this type of learning are: (1) the quality of personal involvement, i.e. the whole person, in both his feeling and cognitive aspects, takes part *in* the learning event; such learning is also (2) self-initiated, (3) pervasive, and (4) evaluated by the learner, in terms of whether the learning is leading toward what he wants to know, whether it illuminates the dark area of ignorance he is experiencing. It is such learning which would seem to be of the essence in learning to nurse. Rogers' principles of learning, abstracted from his own experience, the experience of colleagues and from research, are outlined below:

He contends:

1. human beings have a natural potentiality for learning
2. significant learning takes places when the subject matter is perceived by the student as having relevance for his own purposes
3. learning which involves a change in self organisation — in the perception of oneself — is threatening and tends to be resisted
4. those learnings which are threatening to the self are more easily perceived and assimilated when external threats are at a minimum
5. when threat to the self is low, experience can be perceived in differentiated fashion and learning can proceed
6. much significant learning is acquired through doing
7. learning is facilitated when the student participates responsibly in the learning process
8. self-initiated learning which involves the whole person of

the learner — feelings as well as intellect — is the most lasting and pervasive

9. independence, creativity, and self-reliance are all facilitated when self-criticism and self-evaluation are basic, and evaluation by others is of secondary importance

10. the most socially useful learning in the modern world is the learning of the process of learning, a continuing openness to experience and incorporation into oneself of the process of change.   (Rogers, 1969, pp. 157–163)

EXPERIENTIAL LEARNING APPLIED IN NURSING

A natural potential for learning

Rogers' principles of learning were the foundation upon which the research experiment described in this book was proposed and subsequently designed. These principles seem particularly apposite to nurse education and training, in which the rationale must surely be to build upon, and around, the students' natural desire to learn about nursing, and where better for student nurses than in the ward with the patients? Rogers points out that students are eager to learn, and curious, unless their curiosity is blunted by the system of education, and it may be just such a 'blunting' process which is seen in the change which in some cases takes place between the eager Introductory Block students' questioning and the less than enthusiastic learners who return to a second period in the college of nursing. Learning, as he states, is not always easy, can indeed be painful, but given suitable conditions the students' potential and desire for learning can be released. With regard to his second principle, nursing can hardly be in a more advantageous position, as there must be few students who enter into the course simply aiming to 'get by' — the majority are learning to nurse because they really want to learn how to care for people in need, therefore the process of giving that care is seen as highly relevant to their purposes, and should result in significant learning.

Learning which is resisted

The conflicting values and standards between school and ward are relevant to Rogers' third principle of learning. Perhaps it is inevitable that the somewhat idealised self-image of most 'fledgling nurses' will be threatened on the first encounter with reality in the wards. Perhaps, as Hutty (1965) has said, some of the confusion and difficulties which first year nursing students experience arise because of the students' own failure to adapt — 'they tend to be inflexible in a real situation as opposed to an ideal one' (p. 146). Whatever the reasons, the fact that a threatening situation exists is well known and well researched in nursing — there is considerable evidence that what is expected of the student is different in the two places. The learning which arises from this dilemma has been noted to be unproductive, both in terms of students' attitudes to learning and in regard to standards of patient care (Hunt, 1971). It would seem quite possible that such early experiences may have more far-reaching effects upon the students' view of learning as a life-long process in nursing, an integral part of her professional development as a nurse. It would therefore seem incumbent upon the profession to act by endeavouring to 'ease' the student into the threatening situation with the help of a teacher, in somewhat the way Taylor (1979) described had taken place in Bolton.

Learning climate
The importance of the learning climate in both ward and college is seen when reference is made to Rogers' fourth and fifth principles. Harding (1979) contrasted two metaphorical, but very realistic, ward environments in which 'external threats' were respectively minimal and maximal, and in more serious vein, Fretwell (1979), Ogier (1980) and Orton (1980) have examined the learning environments of the practice areas for nurses. Heath (1979) describes a climate conducive to learning as one in which 'the learner can take risks (in the sense of trying out new behaviours), admit to difficulties and problems, give and receive feedback and cope with allied stress.' The attaining of such an environment is not easy, in particular in a busy ward, and unless staff, teachers and students are able to be mutually supportive the new environment may constitute a threat in a different way.

Significant learning acquired through doing
To place a student in direct experiential confrontation with practical problems, with ethical problems and with personal issues is Rogers' sixth principle, one which he considers one of the most effective ways of promoting learning. It is this principle which is central to the research experiment herein reported, that student nurses be confronted, and involved in coping with the day-to-day problems of nursing — problems and situations which they would experience throughout their nursing training, and that they learn ways of nursing by doing nursing. Indeed all the other principles are subsumed within the participative, active learning situation in which the experimental group student is placed. Although under supervision,

she is free to carry out nursing care orders in her own style, to think through appropriate solutions to individual patient's problems, and to evaluate her decisions and her work in a way which is not possible within a task-oriented work environment. Most of all, the principle of learning to learn was important. Nursing, if it is to survive as a profession, must develop individuals who can not only face the challenge of change, but can capitalise upon it and see the potential where it exists for the improvement of standards of patient care.

The teacher as facilitator
As might be expected, the role of the teacher in Rogers' view is not dissimilar to the role Maslow put forward; only the terminology is different. Rogers describes the teacher as a 'facilitator of learning' — one who is responsible for setting the mood or climate of the learning experience, and who is able to permit learners a sense of freedom to work as they wish, which means accepting that some will be dependent and need direction while others will want much less guidance. The facilitator should not only make as wide a range of learning resources available as is possible in his circumstances, but should actively involve him/herself with the students as they learn, i.e. be a resource person. It would seem a very demanding and difficult role as he must also be capable of realising his own limitations, in that freedom can be granted to students only to the extent that the facilitator is comfortable with it — no easy task indeed, as Boydell (1976) pointed out very clearly when contrasting the role of the traditional versus the participative instructor. Boydell identified one of the early problems, in setting the climate for such autonomous learning, as related to the difficulties learners experienced in defining their own needs: 'most learners arrive expecting all the characteristics of a 'traditional' course' (p. 52). He was here referring to adult learners, not young school children and his statement could be equally true of learners in nursing. There is a connotation of passivity, and a certain peace and orderliness in the traditional conception of learning which is absent from the turbulent changing scene of meaningful, experiential learning advocated by writers such as Rogers and Boydell. The latter described 'experiential learning' in terms which denoted active involvement of the learner in making sense of what he had learned by internally sorting things out for himself so as to gain insight or learning.

The essence, then, of experiential learning is:
(a) problem situation;

(b) sorting things out;
(c) action planning — implications of what has been learned.
   (p. 25)

Such could be said to be the essence of individualised patient care, or equally, on smaller scale, the thinking approach to any task within patient care. It could also constitute a description of the extremely topical concept in nursing — the process of nursing.

Boydell noted four components in the 'learning from work experience' system: the individual, the formal learning structures, the opportunities to learn and the learning climate; and these are, significantly, areas of concern, and of action, in nursing today.

However, the concern of this chapter is with learning, and quite clearly, individual students will differ in the extent to which they are able to learn from their experiences, a fact of which many present day 'facilitators' are aware. Boydell equates the characteristics of the effective learner with those of the self-actualising individual — 'therefore, in order to improve the extent to which individuals are going to be able to learn from their experiences, they must be helped to acquire these self-actualisation characteristics/abilities.' (p. 68)

MEANINGFUL LEARNING

However, all individuals are so different, and the importance of individual differences in learning have been alluded to previously in this text. Students bring with them to the learning scene, their differing abilities and perceptions and expectations. Ausubel, in the frontispiece of his book *Educational Psychology: A Cognitive View* (1968) stresses the importance of recognising and working with such individual differences:

> The most important single factor influencing learning is what the learner already knows. Ascertain this and teach him accordingly.

Ausubel too, is concerned to explain meaningful learning. He identified two dimensions or stages of the learning process. The first was concerned with the ways in which information to be learned was made available to the learner, and the second with the ways in which the learner dealt with the information. Ausubel & Robinson (1969) consider information can be made available in two ways — either the entire content to be learned is presented, given to the student in final form, which they call 'reception learning', or alternatively, only part of what is to be learned is given to the student, and the remainder he must find out, actively seek, by himself. This they term 'discovery learning'. In the second stage, what the learner attempts to do with the information in order to recall it later, may also take two forms. The student may simply attempt to memorise the new material, or he may try to relate the new material to what he already knows, in which case, in Ausubel & Robinson's opinion, meaningful learning occurs.

As the relating process can be applied to material received by reception or discovery learning, it would appear that meaningful learning is not the function of any one particular teaching method or approach. Although such learning is a very individual process, it can be aided, facilitated by the provision of 'subsumers' and 'advance organisers'. These writers consider that in meaningful learning new information is assimilated into the learners' cognitive structure by a process of subsumption, i.e. the new fact or idea is related to existing material in such a way that both are modified and both are given meaning. Through subsumption, new material is anchored to the existing material in the individual's cognitive structure and this anchoring gives the new information stability, i.e. resistance to forgetting. Thus, meaningful learning is dependent upon what is already known, upon a sufficiency of hooks on which to hang the new information (James, quoted in Munn, 1966). Ausubel contends that if an existing set of relevant ideas is not present in the learners' cognitive structure, the only alternative he has is rote learning (Ausubel, 1975,).

To encourage meaningful learning, the teacher should provide suitable advance organisers, i.e. introductory material at a very general level, whose relevance to subsequent learning should be made explicit to students. The function of such organisers is to bridge the gap between what the learner already knows and what he needs to know before he can successfully learn the task in hand, or alternatively to provide subsumers, or hooks, to aid the assimilation of meaningful learning.

The structuring of the learning experience in the research experiment was such that new and general information about the disease process, and medical and nursing problems of patients with gastrointestinal conditions was presented to students prior to their learning of the nursing care of such patients. Thus what were, in the main, lectures by medical and nurse teaching staff, were intended to act as subsumers and advance organisers which would promote anchorage of subsequent specifically relevant material still to be presented.

TRANSFER OF LEARNING

One of the main purposes behind the promotion of such meaningful learning was that it should be capable of use, of transfer from one situation in nursing to another. Such transfer of learning is a prime purpose of much formal education and it is said to occur when a person's learning in one situation influences his learning and performance in other situations. That such transfer does not occur automatically or easily is evidenced by the universality of the debate about lack of integration of theory and practice, which is, in part at least, a debate about a learning problem — the inability of students to relate knowledge gained by instruction to actual work performance.

Transfer may be negative or positive. It is negative when learning or the performance of a task interferes with the learning or performing of another task — a concept akin to that of pro- and retroactive inhibition, and it is positive when learning in one situation is helpful to learning or the solution of problems in a different situation. It should be noted that neither positive nor negative transfer can occur if the student does not perceive the learning in the first situation as in any way related to the second situation. This is one of the points made by Wong, in discussing the difficulties experienced by nursing students in transferring classroom learning to clinical practice. She states:

> ideal transfer demands the students' conscious realization that transfer is possible. (And later) Students need to be committed to the belief that particular facts learned in the classroom study are pertinent in other situations. (Wong, 1979)

Gagné (1970) identified two kinds of transfer which he considered were of importance in education. Lateral transfer he considered took place when an individual was able to perform tasks which, though not identical to a previously learned task were very similar to what had been directly learned and of approximately the same level of complexity, whereas vertical transfer implied a process of building upon past learning in order to attain knowledge and understanding of more advanced concepts and higher-order principles. Although Gagné felt that not a great deal was known about the innate, or internal and individual factors in the promotion of both types of transfer, he considered both were promoted if the initial learning was practised in as wide a variety of situations as possible, and if basic principles were thoroughly learned before proceeding to more advanced learning.

In these views, the elements of earlier theories about transfer of learning are evident. The earliest theory, prominent for many centuries, was the formal discipline theory. It was contended that general exercise of the faculties of the mind, in particular in studying such subjects as Greek, Latin and mathematics, would result in a strengthening of the individual's ability to think and reason. Elements of this theory are extant today, but Thorndike, of stimulus-response fame, produced conclusive evidence in the early Twenties, after research involving the records of more than 13 000 high school students, which disproved the formal discipline theory (Thorndike, 1924). He replaced it with his own, the identical elements theory, which, as might be expected from his adherence to the stimulus-response concept of learning, assumed that identical elements must be present in both the initial learning situation and the one to which transfer occurred. Although this was a much narrower perspective, it did result in the introduction into school curricula of many more practical and socially useful subjects, for example typing and shorthand, woodwork and machine work. However in its very precision lay its downfall, in that it was then, and is even more so today, very difficult to forecast the precise skills and subjects which students will need for their future work. At the same time as Thorndike propounded his theory, there were others who emphasised a contrasting interpretation of transfer named generalisation theory (Judd, 1939). Judd was perhaps the best-known advocate of the latter theory. He believed, as did many others, that the important condition for transfer was for the student to learn general rules or principles, which could then be transferred or generalized to new situations. Judd's theory, and a similar though more comprehensive view, termed transposition theory, were very close to the Gestalt view of transfer. However the difference lay in that the two former failed to take account of the learner's desire to use an insight he had already gained, and this was a vital element in Gestalt transfer theory. Bigge (1971) sets forth some of their beliefs:

> A person is in the best frame of mind for transfer to occur when he is aware of acquiring meanings and abilities that are widely applicable in learning and living...A person must also want to solve new problems, or approach new situations in the light of the insights gained through previous experience... For transfer to occur individuals must generalize — perceive common factors in different situations (and) comprehend them as applicable and appropriate to both, and thereby understand how the generalization can be used...Transfer of learning to

new tasks will be better if, in learning, the learner can discover relationships for himself, and if he has opportunities to apply his learning to a variety of tasks. (p. 273)

THE DIFFICULT INSTRUCTIONAL MOMENT

The role of the teacher as one who supports his students is seen by Perry (1975) as relevant in situations where the knowledge to be taught is contextual and relative, rather than consisting mainly of facts, with their connotations of right or wrong. In fact, he sees as a difficult instructional moment for students, and also for their teachers, the point at which the students' conception of knowledge as a 'quantitative accretion of discrete rightnesses' changes to a conception of knowledge as 'the qualitative assessment of contextual observations and relationships'. From this point onwards, the students' task becomes more integrational and that of the teacher less atomistic.

There seems little doubt that much of the knowledge required for nursing is contextual and relative. Perhaps in the very early stages, there may be, at least in the mind of the student, an overabundance of facts — what Henderson (1966) has called 'an early lethal dose of technology'. If this dose is not diluted for the beginning student with opportunities to see the facts applied in practice, put together to form a whole in the care of a patient, her progress as a learner may be hindered for a long time to come. Could it be that it is the 'difficult instructional moment' which Perry describes, which occurs for many student nurses, on their return to college from practical experience, to undertake their second period of theoretical experience, and which can give rise to discontent and difficulties for both student and teacher. It may be that this is a critical stage of development for the student which is neither well-understood, nor, consequently, well-managed by the teachers in nursing, as a result of which, for many students, their perception of learning as a passive process of assimilating knowledge of right and wrong, good and bad in nursing continues throughout training, and does not develop and change, to become an active, integrational process, in which all knowledge and indeed values are seen as relative. It is only from this point on that critical thinking can progress — the type of thinking which is basic to the problem-solving approach to nursing care relevant to individual patient needs.

Perry emphasises the importance of the teacher's task in presenting uncertainties and disagreements within a subject area to the students, and the use of small group tutorials, individual and group project work, and other such non-directive measures involving a co-operative relationship between teacher and student and active learning on the part of the student. Only in this way can a student develop to the stage where he accepts a commitment to learning as an ongoing, unfolding activity, in fact a life-long process, with what Marton has termed a view of learning as 'something they do' and not just 'something that happens to them' (Marton, 1975, p. 130).

LEARNERS' APPROACHES TO LEARNING

Of recent years, the focus of research into learning, especially learning in higher or further education, has been upon the ways in which students process information presented to them for learning. According to Gagné (1971) such information processing has become the framework within which modern theories of learning have been formulated.

Global or step-by-step learners
Pask (1969), who has worked a great deal in this area, began some of his experiments by simply setting a learning task before a group of 16 students in his laboratory, and then observing what they did with it. This close observation, and an ingenious teach-back testing technique (Pask & Scott, 1972), which has more than a hint of the Skinnerian about it, led them to depict two main types of learner — the 'holists or global learners and serialists or step-by-step learners'. The latter group 'learn, remember and recapitulate a body of information in terms of string-like cognitive structures where items are related by simple data links . . . (and) are intolerant of irrelevant information unless, as individuals, they are equipped with an unusually large memory capacity. Holists, on the other hand, learn, remember and recapitulate as a whole.' The writers also identified two sub-categories of holist — those 'irredundant holists' whose image contained only relevant and essential constituents, and 'redundant holists' whose images contained material derived from data used to enrich the curriculum, i.e. somewhat irrelevant items. Pask, who had set up linear teaching programmes based upon the two different learning strategies, also experimented by 'matching' these programmes with the two different learning styles. In 'matched' groups, serialists were taught using serialist programmes, and holists with holist programmes, and in 'mismatched' groups, serialists were taught using holist programmes and *vice versa*. The results of these, and many similar subsequent experiments, Pask reports

and summarises in tabular form in 1976, and these findings unequivocally support his contention, made four years before, that
learning is more effective when students and teaching methods are
matched:

> the experiments show, very clearly indeed, that the rate, qual-
> ity and durability of learning is crucially dependent upon
> whether or not the teaching strategy is of a sort which suits the
> individual. (Pask & Scott, 1972)

Thus, he states, not that no learning will take place if styles and
strategies of learning are mismatched, but that learning will be less
than it might be.

Green (1974) who entertains such a matching possibility in a
comprehensive study of student nurses' curricular preferences in a
baccalaureate degree programme in nursing at the University of San
Francisco in the United States, concludes that to group together
students with similar learning preferences — and attendant
teaching methods — could be restrictive rather than helpful to the
development of effective learning, especially if it were to be the predominant approach in a curriculum. Students can learn from sharing experiences which are appreciated in different ways by their
peers, thus broadening their own interest in and appreciation for
different methods of learning and teaching.

The implications for education generally and for nurse education
seem to be that a mix of teaching methods is essential if both types
of student are to be catered for and to learn effectively.

Deep and surface-level processing by learners
Marton & Säljö (1976), in Scandinavia, contemporaries of Pask in
London, have also studied differences in process and outcome in
learning, but specifically in relation to the content which was to be
learned. Their work, they considered, was concerned with
'meaningful learning in the true sense of this term' (p. 10), because
they sought out what meaning different students attached to
identical passages or content to be learned.

They stated:

> different students obviously learn different things from one
> and the same text and their knowledge about various scientific
> principles, methods and ideas varies as regards *what is learned*
> instead of merely differing as regards *how much is learned*.
> (Marton & Säljö, 1976, p. 7)

Such qualitative differences in outcome they consider very likely to reflect corresponding differences in process, or the way people set about learning. Their premise is that there are basically two levels of processing — deep-level, in which 'the student is directed towards the intentional content of the learning material' (what is signified), i.e. what the author wants to say, or principles; and surface-level in which 'the student directs his attention towards learning the text itself' (the sign), i.e. a reproductive conception of learning which means the student is more or less forced to keep to a rote-learning strategy. Superficially this may seem just an extension of understanding versus rote, but it may be more than that, in that the meaning assigned to the same content was different for students who used the different levels of processing.

The influence of examinations

As a result of further experimentation, which they admit they found complicated to analyse, Martin & Säljö (1976a) showed the influence of tests and examinations on the students' levels of processing. The levels were not immutable, in that students would alter them in anticipation of a particular type of recall or test. It was fairly obvious that most students anticipated an emphasis on detail in tests, and modified their processing accordingly. In general it appeared that anticipation of an objective test focused their attention on details — 'signs', whereas an essay or oral test appeared to suggest general principles or main points 'what is signified'. Miller & Parlett (1974) categorised students in terms of their behaviour in regard to seeking out cues or hints about forthcoming examinations. Many students appeared to consider that success in examinations was obtained simply by hard work and seemed unaware of any benefits to be gained in 'picking up hints'. Such students they termed 'cue-deaf'. Others were aware that it could be helpful to be perceptive and receptive of any clues — they were 'cue-conscious', and still others deliberately sought out staff and in general acted very positively in their search for information which might be helpful in passing examinations — they were 'cue-seekers'. Such information as they could glean strongly influenced their preparatory study and work. It has of course been known for some considerable time that students are influenced by what they anticipate in examinations (Silvey, 1951). Indeed, although Miller & Parlett's work was done with final year Honours students in university, there must be few teachers, in nursing or general education, who are unaware of the phenomenon of cue-seeking. A brief glimpse at the very well-thumbed folders containing copies of previous examination papers, provided they remain on the shelves to be seen, would corroborate evidence of cue-seeking.

The inherent danger of the examination system, that if trivia are examined then trivia will be learned, is brought into focus again with Marton & Säljö's work. The dependent variable may be, for many students, the independent variable. Marton (1975) states — in regard to his work — 'the idea is simple enough: in order to help the students understand, we must first understand their way of thinking about the topics with which we are concerned.'

How do they think about nursing? Of one thing we can be sure, they will all think slightly differently, but, again with Marton & Säljö: 'it is fundamentally important to recognise the link between the level of processing adopted and the level of understanding reached' (Marton & Säljö, 1976a, p. 123). Many students, in nursing as elsewhere, are capable of using 'deep' or 'surface' strategies. If the current demands of the examination system are such that students, on the whole, adopt a surface approach to the information-processing of the various subjects in their curriculum, then the important meaning may be lost — the analogy in nursing is clear.

4

Measurement and evaluation

INTRODUCTION

Student nurses, in common with students the world over, as indeed with students through the ages, are examined, tested, measured and assessed. Increasingly, of recent years, their education and training programmes have been, and are evaluated.

This chapter contains a brief overview of measurement and evaluation in education. Although similar in meaning, the two terms are not synonymous. Evaluation is used, in general, with a more global connotation, encompassing measurement within its sphere. The former is also a much more recent arrival on the educational scene, which was dominated, especially in the early part of this century, by an emphasis on the measurement of differences between individuals. Stanley & Hopkins (1972), and many other writers, equate measurement with tests — tests of achievement, intelligence, interest, aptitude — and the construction, administration and scoring of such tests or examinations. Evaluation they consider to be a related procedure, concerned with interpreting such scores, saying whether they are good or bad for a specific purpose — a summing-up process in which value judgements play a large part. Cronbach (1977) states that 'evaluation is not just testing ... (it) is the process of judging whether or not the goals of schooling are being attained by the individual, the class, or the school system' (p. 683).

The first part of this chapter is about tests, or examinations (the terms are used interchangeably) and the second part is about evaluation.

TESTS AND MEASUREMENT

Student nurses spend a considerable amount of their time taking tests, both objectives tests and essay type tests, and presumably a certain amount of time preparing for them. Their teachers take

52

time constructing tests and marking them. Part of the evaluation of this research experiment was dependent upon scores on objective tests and essays. Finally and most importantly, no student nurse can become a registered nurse unless she has successfully completed the Final State examination set by the General Nursing Council. In England and Wales, since 1977 this has incorporated an essay-type test and an objective test. In Scotland it is of an essay format. Qualification as a registered nurse is not entirely dependent upon written tests. The student nurse must also obtain satisfactory ward assessments and reports, but this particular form of assessment was not dealt with in this research nor is it the subject of this chapter.

Origins and characteristics

Measurement and evaluation are inseparable from the process of learning, and it is fascinating to study the almost parallel progress and changing emphases in these two closely related subject areas. Just as the historical origins of learning are lost in antiquity, so too are the origins of testing and measurement. An elaborate system of civil service examinations existed in China several centuries before Christ (Du Bois, 1966). The ancient Greeks used testing as a part of their educational process and the Socratic method of interspersing instruction with oral testing still is used today in many classrooms. The researches of Haley (1977), although dependent on an oral transmission of historical facts, strongly suggest that Kunta Kinte, and his kafo mates, in mid-18th century in a small village deep within Africa were a part of an organised system of education which culminated in an oral and written examination for these young students of the arafang.

The modern era of a more scientific precision in measurement is presaged by the writings and work of Fisher, Galton and E. L. Thorndike, who, among many others at the turn of the century, brought about a relegation of the oral examination — its place taken by the written test and, even then, a few of these were objective tests. The very first known use of the objective test was by the English schoolmaster, the Reverend George Fisher in 1864 (Stanley & Hopkins, 1972).

Following on from the work of the early pioneers of testing, two very broad groups of tests could be distinguished. The standardised tests, of which there are now so many that massive compendia are produced regularly, and whole departments in universities exist purely in order to deal with test-related matters, had their origins in the intelligence tests established by Binet in 1904 in France. These tests have developed to include not only measurement in the cognitive domain, but also in the affective and psychomotor domains. A great variety of 'instruments', as such tests are often called, exist to measure achievement, motivation, interests, aptitude and manual dexterity. In tandem with standardised tests, and just as extensively used, have been the tests and examinations devised by teachers, concerned to regularly assess the progress of their students. These tests, which have considerable impact on the daily lives of students in all types of courses, remain for the most part, unpublished, perhaps why they have been termed 'fugitive instruments' (Goodwin & Klausmeier, 1975, p. 493). Textbooks, and courses, instruct teachers in all matters relevant to the compilation, scoring and use of such tests.

So much emphasis on testing must be to some purpose. Vernon (1940) states 'examinations have far too great a burden to bear' (p. 276). Intelligence tests, vocabulary tests, are frequently used to predict future ability to cope with and succeed in a variety of educational settings and courses. Teacher-made tests, as opposed to nationally standardised tests, regulate pupil entry to certain courses and classes in school, which in turn regulates the pupil's preparation and submission for national examinations which in turn has considerable influence upon his or her future career prospects. The General Nursing Council (Scotland) use a standardised test to permit entry to nurse training for prospective students who do not have the requisite Ordinary or Higher Grade certificates.

Norm-referenced and criterion-referenced tests

Popham (1978), in inimitable style, distinguishes between 'sort-'em-out-and-spot-the-best' tests, and 'criterion-referenced measurement', which latter type he considers 'the most exciting measurement contender to trot down the testing trail' (p. 8) in recent years. He states:

> When a testing system is directed toward the isolation of examinees' relative standings with respect to each other, it is perfectly satisfactory as long as all one needs to know is who is better (or worse) than whom. But if one tries to apply such a relatively oriented testing system to settings in which one must know precisely what it is that examinees can or can't do, then such a testing system comes up short. That is where the educational testing situation is today. (p. 9)

That too would seem to be where the testing situation in the system of nursing education is today.

The credit for creating a solution to the test dilemma, Popham gives to Glaser, who introduced the expressions norm-referenced and criterion-referenced measurement (Glaser, 1963). The former discerned an examinee's relative standing, i.e. graded him in some way, the latter identified his mastery, or non-mastery, of 'specific behaviours'.

Criterion-referenced tests were a natural development from the rising interest in programmed learning and the necessity to firstly specify precisely-worded behavioural objectives (cf. Mager, 1962) and then to test whether or not these objectives had been achieved by the learner. Thus the relative standing of students *vis-à-vis* each other faded in significance, to be replaced by an absolute measure as to which objectives the student had, or had not attained. Ebel (1979) explains the criterion as the attainment of the objectives of the particular learning experience, whereas the norm is the achievement of some specified group of students on a test. Both types of tests have essentially the same job to do, i.e. to measure achievement in learning. The individual test questions used in the two may well be identical, but the purpose of the norm-referenced test is to *indicate* a student's degree of success in learning and of the criterion-referenced test to *ensure* that certain things will be learned (Ebel, 1979, p. 11).

McGaghie (1978) discusses the same concept in regard to medical education. Mastery learning he equates with competence as defined by the educational objective — and he further stated that different levels of mastery or competence existed and should therefore be distinguished and tested at the different stages of the learning process — a mattter of current concern and relevance for nursing assessment. McGaghie considers examinations to be among the least understood and most misused tools of education, used mainly to 'grade on the curve' (p. 69) a clear reference to norm-referencing, rather than to indicate mastery or otherwise of competencies necessary to safe practice.

The notion of a normal curve is basic to any consideration of norm-referenced tests. Individual students are placed in position on a scale, usually compiled from the scores of a 'norm' group, i.e. other students who have taken the same test, or, in the case of some national and standardised tests, on the scores of individuals considered similar in age, I. Q., or other category. A normal distribution is shown in Figure 1.

As most educational variables have been shown to be distributed normally in the population, early test constructors aimed to produce tests which retained that normal distribution. Such tests,

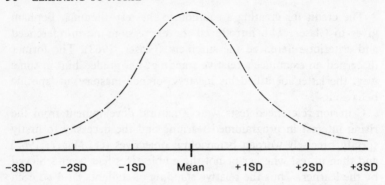

Note: Deviations from the mean are marked off in units of standard deviation (SD). 68% of the area under the curve lies between + ISD and − ISD from the mean

Fig. 1 The 'normal distribution'

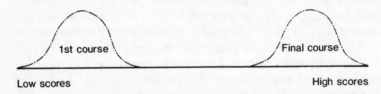

Fig. 2 A continuum of proficiency (adapted from Popham, 1978)

administered following a specific learning experience, gave evidence of progress by simply shifting every student further up on a continuum as can be seen in Figure 2 (adapted from Popham, 1978). In other words, students entered normally distributed and went out, at the end of their learning, normally distributed. However, that entire conception was threatened, if not upended in criterion-referenced testing and the step-by-step processes of programme learning, where clear objectives have been set, instruction has been geared to the specific achievement of these objectives and the test tests that achievement or otherwise by the testee, i.e. the absolute not the relative. The typical pre- and post-instruction curve, if instruction has been effective, then assumes a shape quite different from the normal curve, and similar to Figure 3. Although it is possible that all three Figures relate to standardised scores, it is nonetheless interesting to compare the curve in Figure 3 with the histograms in Appendix B, related to the objective test administered in this research, and the findings in relation to the essay type of test, and to conjecture just what it is the two different types of test may be measuring . . .?

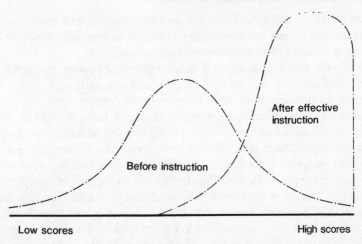

Fig. 3 Distribution 'before and after effective instruction' (Popham, 1978)

The test controversy

Criticisms of tests and testing are, and always have been, rife. Tests are said to measure only superficial, unimportant aspects of achievement; to 'label' students as bright or dull, thus in either case distorting their expectations and diminishing their efforts; to place students under stress, exposing them to unnecessary experience of failure; to destroy confidence; to kill the joy of learning; to carry cultural and middle-class bias, and to force teachers into a restrictive position described as 'teaching to the test' (Ebel, 1979). The latter disapprobation is of a teacher spending considerable time in preparing students to handle specific questions likely to be included in tests, at the expense, it is inferred, of more educationally desirable goals, such as encouraging freedom in learning, discovery, and problem-solving.

However, the foremost problems and criticisms of tests of all types are in regard to their reliability and validity, which two key concepts Pilliner (1973) defines very clearly and in succint detail, although only his initial definitions are quoted here:

> Reliability is 'the extent to which a test gives consistent results' ... Validity is 'the extent to which a test actually measures the entity which it was designed to measure'. (pp. 52/53)

Objective test or essay

These twin concepts of reliability and validity are frequently at the root of debates about the two most commonly used tests of achievement, both in general education and in nursing education, i.e. the objective or multiple-choice test and the essay-type of test. These two types of test are often also considered to represent almost the opposite poles of an objective/subjective continuum.

To the extent that any test score reflects the private, subjective, unverifiable impressions and values of any one particular scorer, it must be deficient both in meaning and usefulness to either the student or the institution requiring evidence of his achievement. As the name would indicate, there is considered to be more objectivity in multiple-choice tests than in essay tests. The former can test a wider range of objectives and knowledge; questions are generally much more precisely formulated, thus less ambiguous of interpretation; 'bluffing' in answering is reduced (not eliminated, as guessing is always possible); scoring is completely reliable, and, especially if done by computer, not subject to human vagary. The fact that subjectivity plays its part in the selection of content to be examined in an objective test, and in the fact that students may come to such tests in a variety of moods and motivation, is almost disregarded in the general approval of the reliability of the marking and the fact that the individual test items can be subjected to various types of item analysis.

The marking of essay scripts
It is the issue of reliability in marking which is most often raised by critics of the essay type of test. The definitive work in this respect is that of Hartog & Rhodes in 1936 in Britain. In two books, published in the same year, they thoroughly investigated the marking of essay scripts, and the whole subject of variability in such marking, and showed that, no matter which method, i.e. analytical (marking key) or impression marking, was employed, marks of individual examiners varied widely. Not only did different examiners differ in their standards of marking, but individual markers differed when they re-marked a script they had marked on a previous occasion. Hartog & Rhodes studied marks awarded for scripts submitted in English examinations, and also scripts submitted in subjects such as chemistry, mathematics and foreign languages. Thus, there is no reason to suppose their comments and findings other than also applicable to the marking of scripts in nursing examinations. These early writers suggested the use of teams of markers, whose marks could be aggregated, then averaged, as one way to reduce unreliability of marking and its consequences in the erroneous failure or passing of candidates. This system of teams of markers was adopted in the marking of essay scripts in this research project.

Some years later, Finlayson (1951) and Wiseman (1949) wrote on the subject of reliability in essay marking, repeating and elaborating upon some of the earlier experiments of Hartog & Rhodes (1936). Finlayson argued that reliability of essays was not just a matter of consistency of marking, but included the variability of the examinees from day to day, and variability in the essay topics, whether in fact different topics could be considered as measuring the same ability day by day. Wiseman, who was discussing the marking of English composition essays, appeared to be in favour of general impression markers rather than analytical markers. With the latter he felt that the best essay might not be at the top of the list because the total Gestalt was more than the sum of its parts. It may seem that this present discussion is not particularly relevant to the examination of nursing, and yet the problem of many markers of Final State scripts is whether to score each detail, i.e. use a marking key, or to take a general impression, i.e. the total Gestalt. Some of the Final State examination questions lend themselves to the analytical framework approach to marking, whereas others, which for example, ask examinees to discuss the care of a terminally ill patient, lend themselves much more to a Gestalt approach in marking.

What does the essay test?

In general, the view of these two main types of test above discussed, is that whereas the objective test can test a wide range of knowledge linked to specific objectives, the especial advantage of essays is their potential for testing 'the student's abilities to organize, integrate and synthesize his knowledge, to use his information to solve novel problems and to be original or innovative in his approaches to problem situations' (Thorndike & Hagen, 1977, p. 269). Mehrens & Lehmann (1978) make very similar claims, while pointing out that simply writing a question in essay format does not guarantee that such qualities will be tapped. The major difficulties which are inherent in phrasing essay questions in order to tap such abilities as above referred to are recognised by many educators. However, most of the debate is taken up with the as yet unresolved problem of how to assess the student's answer in a less subjective way.

The close subjective link between question and answer was amusingly, yet tellingly, recounted by Stalnaker, in a scholarly, somewhat prosaic publication on the subject of educational measurement. Stalnaker (1951) wrote:

> Years ago, one of the possible theme titles on a College Board English paper was 'The Vanishing Horse'. The examiners had

in mind an essay of a more or less economic kind on the disappearance of horses with the coming of the motor car. But the readers found that not a few students accepted the title as a challenge to create a fairy story, and one theme with an improved title, 'Rudolph, the Vanishing Horse', will never be forgotten by those fortunate enough to peruse it. Needless to say, it was found to be almost impossible to grade on the same scale used for the sober accounts of the disappearance of quadrupeds as prime movers. (p. 520)

One would tend to consider nursing examinations so very different from the above, in that they require much more precise answers, as a result of asking much more precise questions. Yet, if we encourage a problem-solving individualised approach in the practice of nursing can we expect, indeed look for, an essentially factual sameness in replies to questions, especially if we use essay questions for presumably the very purposes which Thorndike & Hagen have put forward?

Consider what may be an adequate answer to the under-noted questions, set by teachers in two different colleges, for end of course examinations for students who participated in this research:

(a) A young woman, recently engaged, is in your ward recovering from surgical treatment for ulcerative colitis. Describe the special care required for this patient in whom ileostomy has been performed. What psychological problems may present in this patient and how could you as a nurse, help overcome these problems?

and

(b) Describe the management of a patient with ulcerative colitis following surgery for this condition.

Is the answer which will certainly pass, and, if grading is the system, will gain better marks, a sober and accurate list of appropriate procedures and observations in post-operative care; or is it an imaginative account, entitled in the first case — 'How the nurse helped Mary and Bill face their future', or alternatively 'Facing Life Together, with a Stoma as well' — and in the second 'Was there a Stoma, and if so where, what type and why?' It is interesting to speculate how a Final State examiner would have marked the two different types of script — whether a marking key or impression marker would have scored the imaginative or the prosaic higher.

The problem is of course neither so clearly dichotomous nor so extreme as has been depicted, but it is possibly difficulties similar to this which led the General Nursing Council (England and Wales) to change over to an objective type of test for the Final State examination prior to Registration. The reasons Holden, reported by Thompson (1979), gave for the change over were in order to cover a wider range of topics within the syllabus of training, to attempt to overcome question-spotting which leads inevitably to 'pat' answers, but especially because it was virtually impossible to achieve any measure of reliability in the marking of essay questions. He contended:

> that markers agree on the order of superiority of a batch of papers, but disagree widely in the actual marks they give — which is critical around the pass mark of a pass/fail exam. (p. 29)

Holden's interview in the nursing press was occasioned by the outcry which the switch to multiple choice tests from essays had engendered — a torrent of complaints which came not only from student nurses, but also from their teachers. The General Nursing Council (England and Wales) opinion that the change brought about a fairer system of examination was quite clearly not shared by many of the examinees.

What should we measure?

Just what it is either type of test is measuring, no one is quite sure, and all concerned have their own subjective views. At least in nursing, written tests are not the only measure of nursing competence, although such tests occupy an important place.

The choice and use of different testing techniques is closely related to the ends those techniques are designed to serve, which is of course related to the conundrum of what it is we wish to measure in nursing examinations. Pilliner (1977) stated:

> What might be called the 'truth' about an educational system can most readily be discovered by a hard look at the examination procedures it engenders. (p. 14)

That 'hard look' could well be said to be taking place in nursing education today, but — as said St Augustine around the year AD400:

> For so it is, O Lord my God, I measure it;
> but what it is that I measure I do not know.
>
> (St Augustine's Lament)

EVALUATION

What it is: A changing emphasis

Evaluation is concerned with the making of value judgments, not, as Suchman (1977) pointed out, regardless of an informed basis for such judgment, but making use of scientific method to collect data concerning the degree to which some specified activity achieves some desired effect. At present, in nursing literature, the word is predominantly used in connection with the final stage of the nursing process, i.e. the stage at which the student (or trained nurse) should stand apart and assess the worth of her nursing intervention. Although evaluation in this sense was a part of the learning experience of the experimental group students in this research project, it is evaluation in its wider sense which is the subject of the next few pages, evaluation as concerned with programmes, curricula, or units of learning experience. This is the view of evaluation adopted by the Joint Board of Clinical Nursing Studies, in their 'Course Evaluation Package' issued in 1978:

> In evaluation the spotlight is on gathering information about, and judging the *course*, rather than the individual *student* as is the case in assessment. (p. 1) (Author's italics)

Green & Stone (1977) define evaluation not dissimilarly:

> Evaluation is the systematic documentation of the consequences of programmes and the determination of their worth in order to make decisions about them. (p. 4)

Green & Stone, in questioning the purposes of evaluation, allude to some of its many uses: is it to measure (test), to prove (present evidence), to improve (change), to judge (determine value), to advocate (take a position), to illuminate (discover facts or 'the truth')? That it may, at differing times, be some or all of these things depends to a certain extent upon the people to whom it is addressed, or, in some cases, who have requested it, for example the policy makers, the teachers, the students. This very broad view of the possible functions of evaluation is in line with the views of Miller & Parlett (1974), advocates of the illuminative evaluation approach — the approach adopted within the research described in this book, and referred to in more detail in Chapter 5. The characteristics of illuminative evaluation they consider to be that it is problem-centred — beginning with issues and concerns as defined in real life settings: it is practitioner-oriented — its main function to provide information for educators; it is cross-disciplinary; methodologically eclectic and heuristically organised. By the latter statement, the writers mean that as a study unfolds, the researcher progressively focuses and redefines the areas of inquiry as crucial issues are uncovered.

It is interesting that all four authors referred to above advocate such an all-encompassing approach — what might be called the approach of the Seventies — and which contrasts so sharply with the so-called Tylerian approach of the Forties, when the emphasis was on the evaluation of specific and behaviourly stated objectives (Tyler, 1942). According to Harlen (1976), a line of development in evaluation strategies can be traced: 'the changes to more widely based data gathering being brought about by dissatisfaction with results from information gained more 'scientifically' but more narrowly' (p. 37).

Two main strategies

Process and product

Meleis & Benner (1975) consider that the dynamic changes occurring in higher education today have made necessary a similar dynamism in designing evaluation procedures, and that traditional procedures are no longer adequate. Because evaluation should be responsive to the changing needs of the situation two different types should be considered. They define and compare these two, i.e. process and product evaluation. Process evaluation is a continuous, ongoing evaluation, undertaken as a programme, especially a new and innovatory programme, is in progress, and providing feedback to the educator, to enable her to adjust her teaching strategy or content if thought necessary. Its purpose is to facilitate prompt decision making. Product evaluation is concerned with outcomes. It measures end-products, such as learning gains, and should more appropriately be used when a programme is sufficiently developed to warrant testing. Its purpose is to judge the efficiency and efficacy of a programme, and its use facilitates comparison of the outcomes of two different programmes. While both are important, used inappropriately, the writers consider these two types of evaluation may not only fail to guide decision making but misguide it, i.e. product evaluation used too soon may cause the abandonment of a programme before it has been developed, and process evaluation cannot adequately compare different programmes or answer questions about efficacy or efficiency. The latter type of evaluation, however, has no point unless the results are translated into changes or corrective measures.

The foregoing is very similar to Rowntree's (1974) view of the respective roles of macro- and micro-evaluation. The former assesses the whole, with the aim of benefiting students in some future learning situation, whereas the latter assesses parts of the whole, with the aim of improving on-going teaching for the present students.

Formative and summative
It was just such feedback of evaluative information into a developing programme, or during the intermediate stage of the evolving of a new teaching strategy that Scriven (1967) described as formative evaluation. Summative evaluation was his term for the assessment of a fully-operating programme in its entirety. Scriven also differentiated between the roles and goals of evaluation. Goals he saw as judgments of the worth or success of the programme in achieving that for which it was designed. However, in his opinion, evaluation did not end at that point — it had to be put to use. Its role was therefore to aid in decision-making — as to whether a programme or curriculum should continue, be changed, or cease.

Of goals or goal-free
Scriven further suggested that a programme's effects should be measured independently of whether stated goals were achieved. His goal-free concept of evaluation therefore included the assessment of side-effects or unintended outcomes, as well as of anticipated consequences. How well does the course achieve its goals had become the slogan, Scriven wrote, instead of how good is the course 'but it is obvious if the goals aren't worth achieving then it is uninteresting how well they are achieved' (Scriven, 1967, p. 52). Evaluation of the stated goals he termed intrinsic evaluation, and included in the ambit of this type of evaluation, the course content, grading procedures and teacher attitudes. The effects of all these upon the students, as seen perhaps in differences between pre- and post-tests, between control or experimental groups, on any number of criteria, he called pay-off evaluation. Of pure pay-off evaluation he was very critical, considering its appeal lay in the seeming precision of its results, especially when these were compared with the seeming 'messiness' of results from a thorough intrinsic evaluation. It is interesting that Scriven, writing some five years later, in 1972, has come to stress the unintended outcomes as often of more significance than the goals as such, indeed that for the evaluator to draw any distinction between them was irrelevant. He drew an analogy between the testing of new drugs in medical research, and testing the outcomes of a new educational programme, and suggested that

the investigator should be 'blinded' as in drug trials, i.e. the goals of the programme should not be disclosed to him. Thus, he considers, the investigator will look more carefully for all outcomes, unbiased by whether they were intended or not. Scriven stressed it was the evaluation which should be goal-free, not the curriculum planning. Green & Stone (1977) considered that perhaps the most important aspect of the discussion which followed Scriven's exposition of goalfree evaluation was that it alerted the evaluator to both sides of the coin. Once alerted it was possible that his evaluation design would be such as to be sensitive to both planned and unplanned effects.

Katz (1978) also used the analogy of the drug trial in his 'Guidelines for Evaluating a Training Programme for Health Personnel', in which he states that the evaluator should ask not just does the drug — in this case, the programme work — but how does it work, how long is it effective and what are the side-effects. He too emphasises the wholeness of approach which utilises not just traditional evaluation, i.e. have the objectives of the course been met, but also takes cognisance of the context in which the programme operates, the problems and issues it encounters, the unintended outcomes it produces and what elements facilitate or impede its success. Katz comments upon the uniqueness of every evaluation, and considers that the methodology and overall approach will change with each programme evaluated, as will the role of the evaluator. He, or she may in some cases be viewed as simply a data collector, in others as an agent of change.

Evaluation and research

The association, in the minds of many, between evaluation and change is but one of many features of evaluation which make it seem synonymous with research in education, in particular with action research. Weiss (1972) and Overton & Stinson (1977) discuss 'evaluation research' thus clearly linking the two. Nisbet (1974) considered evaluation an extension of educational research, sharing its roots and using its methods and skills. A definition of educational research which Nisbet & Entwistle (1973) had given a year previously makes the link more explicit:

educational research consists in careful, systematic attempts to understand the educational process and, through understanding, to improve its efficiency. This shift of emphasis from 'understanding' to 'improvement' is likely to be disputed by many who are active in what they claim to be wholly respectable educational research which does not aim at improvement — such as historical studies or comparative education. (p. 113)

Thus it would seem that evaluation, one aim of which is certainly improvement, may be equated with 'not wholly respectable research', but research nonetheless. Peters & White (1973), both philosophers, are precise:

Basic research aims at the development of explanatory theory, action research is concerned with 'on the spot' improvement of current educational practices. (p. 100)

This particular definition seems very close to Scriven's concept of formative evaluation, indeed Scriven uses the two terms — research and evaluation — apparently interchangeably:

formative evaluation — this kind of research is often called process research. (Scriven, 1967, p. 51)

It would seem at times almost simply a matter of semantics, evaluation and research — product and process, summative and formative — Cooper (1976) wonders whether Scriven's stark division into summative and formative is helpful as even revision of a developing programme is bound to have a great deal in it to help anyone making a summative judgment.

Evaluation and nursing

There is evidence, in the increasing number of evaluative studies carried out in the field of nursing education, of the use of both main types of evaluation, and of a certain blurring of the edges between the two. There is also considerable variety of approach, and of scale, in such studies.

Many of the Royal College of Nursing studies of nursing care and research reports are in fact micro-evaluations of the worth of certain curriculum content and teaching strategies in terms of the needs of nursing practice, although the word evaluation may not be present in their titles — in particular the work of Hunt (1974), Birch (1975) and Lamond (1974) are apposite. There are countless other relatively small-scale studies, formative or process in ethos, such as those of Hauf (1975) and Pensivy (1977) which are of value in improving on-going teaching strategies. Tibbitts, et al (1978) in a very careful and statistically-based study, sought to distinguish the relative effectiveness of five different teaching methods in nursing, their criteria of effectiveness solely the students' test scores, both immediately after instruction, and on short- and long-term retention, i.e. three weeks and eleven weeks post-instruction. Hopkins & Wright (1978) on albeit smaller and simpler scale, reported a similar evaluation of teaching methods in basic nursing education and Ogundeyin (1980) looked at the effectiveness of self-instructional units in post-basic nursing education. Bendall's (1973) work on the effectiveness of the examination system is somewhat akin to process evaluation, in that it examined a part of the whole, ongoing system of nurse education and training. This evaluation was very influential in bringing about change in the final nursing examination system in England and Wales.

More breadth of approach is seen in the evaluations of entire programmes in nurse education and training. One of the earliest innovatory nursing programmes in this country, which took account of both goals and unintended outcomes of the intervention was the Glasgow experiment, evaluated by Scott Wright (1961) and previously referred to. Both Scott Wright and Pomeranz (1973), who 'evaluated by research' (p. 19) the experiment at St George's Hospital in London, used several criteria to measure the effects of the experimental programmes, not only upon the students, but upon the other staff involved in the whole undertaking. A little later than the Glasgow experiment, but on the other side of the Atlantic, Allen & Reidy (1971) undertook, and reported, an extremely comprehensive evaluation of the first five years of the first diploma level nursing programme in Canada, which took place at the Ryerson Polytechnical Institute in Toronto. This study was quite explicitly termed evaluation research and was designed 'to permit a flexible approach to an exceedingly complex situation' (p. 3) and to be 'practitioner-oriented', i.e. to provide information and insight for those involved in the process of nursing education, by examining a wide range of criteria. House (1977) in an article, the title of which linked the terms evaluation and research, also stressed the need for the nursing profession to examine more criteria than simply examination results before pronouncing a nursing course worthwhile or otherwise, and proceeded to do so in a subsequent article (House, 1977a), taking account of such matters as student satisfaction with their training, student effectiveness as nurses, achievement motivation, and attrition rates, amongst other factors.

Many of these studies, by including student opinion of various aspects of their education process, highlight the importance of such opinion in evaluation. Beck (1978) considered the point of evaluating achievement was lost if the student did not share in the process and Dagsland (1965) felt evaluation to be the right of the student. Logan & Grosvenor (1972) would seem to be in agreement with both writers referred to above, and indeed with the developing trend in educational evaluation which is directly to involve interested parties.

In many of the studies above referred to, evaluation was not planned into the programme from the outset, as Taba (1962) suggests is necessary. While this is possible, and increasingly done, with new and innovatory programmes, the importance of evaluation of established programmes should not be underplayed. The trend, presaged by the Glasgow experiment, and by the Briggs Report a decade later, and itself in a sense an example of a nationally commissioned evaluation of the ongoing system of the preparation of nurses, is to judge the value of nurse education and training against its ability to meet the changing needs of people and society for nursing. Allen (1977) states that 'the criteria by which we judge anything reflect the prevailing values of the times' (p. 9) and suggests that the critical attributes or criteria for programme development in nursing education today are relevance, relatedness and accountability. She defines these concepts thus:

> Relevance — The extent to which the goals, activities, and outcomes of the nursing educational programme are a response to the needs of a particular community or country...
> Relatedness — The extent to which the parts of the nursing programme, i.e. curriculum, teaching of nursing, practice of nursing and research, and administration, influence each other in developing programme goals and in shaping their achievement...
> Accountability — The extent to which the programme teaches the student nurse that the primary responsibility in nursing is to the patient. (Similarly in teaching, the primary responsibility is to the student). (pp. 10–11)

The swing of the pendulum

It would seem that as the literature, and the techniques of evaluation have proliferated, the *modus operandi* has become more and more complicated. The very comprehensive approach to evaluation, such as is described by Miller & Parlett, is seen by Cox (1979) as an attempt to 'get away from the dangers of reducing a complex process like education to a set of simple behavioural objectives', an approach which she warns may be so all-encompassing a description of one situation as to lead to difficulties of application of what has been learned to another situation. Illuminative evaluation would certainly seem to represent the furthest swing of the pendulum from the somewhat simplistic view represented by the early work on evaluation of Tyler and Mager. However, in spite of the fact that De Landsheere, writing in 1979, criticised Mager as seeming to have forgotten that education concerned the whole person, he (De Landsheere) considered that the concept of objectives is essential to the concept of education, a view which would appear to be shared by Cox, above referred to. De Landsheere explained that to educate means to guide — to guide and nowhere are mutually exclusive — to lead just somewhere is not sufficient — 'the destination of education is by nature positive . . . there can be no "correct" evaluation without clear objectives' (pp. 79–81).

There is no doubt that the destination of education in nursing is positive, and that it can only benefit as a result of both smallscale studies capable of evaluation in terms of relatively simple behavioural objectives, and much larger-scale evaluations of programmes the objectives of which are more complex and which will change and evolve as society's needs for the nurse and nursing change and evolve.

PART 2

Nursing
*An experiment
in integration of theory
and practice*

5

Context and approach

THE SETTING FOR THE RESEARCH

This research took place within the nurse education and training
programme in Scotland. It was conducted within the apprenticeship programme by means of which 96%* of learners are prepared for either Registration or Enrolment, in particular, within
that part of the programme in which student nurses are prepared
for the qualification of Registered General Nurse (RGN), i.e. the
'traditional' College of Nursing and Hospital based programme.
This is the programme in which the student nurses experience:

a theoretical component of 26 weeks in 'Block' or the College of
Nursing, and

a practical component of 118 weeks of nursing in the wards and
departments of the hospital(s)

a total of 144 weeks.

Figure 4 depicts this research setting, and also the subject matter of
the experiment.

The choice of subject for the experimental course was influenced
by a number of equally important points. It should be a part of the
general medical and surgical nursing course in the General Nursing
Council (Scotland) syllabus for RGN training and not a specialist subject such as, for example, obstetrics. There is evidence both in the
literature (Harrison et al, 1977) and in the author's experience, that
specialist subjects tend to be perceived as well-integrated by most
students, whereas general medicine and surgery is perceived as least
well-integrated. The subject should deal, mainly, with common disorders and diseases affecting men and women, and there should be
available, in the different wards, a sufficient number of patients suffering from such diseases so as to make it likely that sufficient relevant experience would be available to the students and their
teachers. In addition, the number of curriculum hours devoted to

* Figure obtained from GNC (Scotland) Quarterly Returns, 1978

73

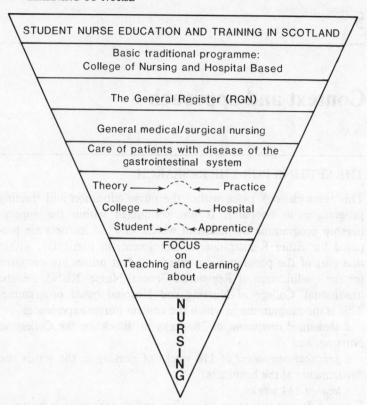

Fig. 4 The setting for the research

the subject should be sufficient to permit some comparison of the treatment with the traditional method of teaching and learning experienced by the student nurses.

Taking all of this into account, the most appropriate subject area in the Syllabus (General Nursing Council (Scotland) 1973) was considered to be that entitled 'Digestive Tract and Abdomen'.

Patients suffering from disease of the digestive system accounted for the highest number of discharges from hospital per 100 000 population in Scotland in the year 1977 (Information Services Division, 1978), and Gribble (1977) drew attention to the very high hospital admission rate for patients with such diseases south of the Border. The majority of these patients are nursed in general medical or surgical wards and thus constitute a fair proportion of the students' nursing work. Not only are a sufficient number of such patients likely to be available for an experiment in nurse education such as envisaged, but especially because of their high numbers it is important that the student should have a thorough understanding of their care.

Investigation revealed that the above subject was usually taught within the first six months of training in the Phase I programme, and prior to any teaching of specialist subjects. Thus, for the student nurse who was meeting this subject matter for the first time in her nursing education, i.e. not the previously trained student nurse, the experimental teaching method would, in a planned and controlled way, link the theory with the practice of nursing of patients with disease of the gastrointestinal tract. It would take the nurse, while she was a student and therefore supernumerary to the ward staff, out from the college and into the ward, as an apprentice together with her teacher, there to be taught and to learn about nursing by giving nursing care.

AIM AND OBJECTIVES

The aim of the study was the facilitation of integration of theory and practice in nursing. The experiment was the means towards the achievement of the aim, and as such had a number of objectives, which are listed below:

1. to help the student nurse integrate theory and practice in nursing;
2. to increase communication between teaching staff and ward nursing staff;
3. to lessen the gap between the ideal and reality in nurse education;
4. to bridge the gap between education and service;
5. to better prepare the student nurse for her ward work and responsibilities;
6. to improve ward staff's understanding of what a student nurse can do at various stages of training;
7. to improve standards of nursing by supervising the student nurse in giving planned and individualised patient care;
8. to diminish stress for the ward teacher by making the student nurse supernumerary;
9. to diminish stress for the teacher by giving a measure of control in the choice of patients and consequently a measure of predictability of teaching;
10. to diminish stress for the student nurse by making her supernumerary while she was giving care and being taught on the ward;

11. to provide an effective learning experience, i.e.
    a. to stimulate students' interest in their studies;
    b. to enable students to take part in class discussions;
    c. to demonstrate learning by means of gain scores on an objective test devised especially for the purpose;
    d. to demonstrate retention of learning by means of scores on the above test;
12. to establish whether differences existed between students taught by the experimental method and those taught by the traditional method in terms of test scores; and
13. to establish whether differences existed between scores of all students in the sample on the objective test referred to above and scores on college-set essay examinations of similar subject matter.

The formulation and use of these objectives were a vital part of the research. Objectives are concerned with communication and evaluation. They helped clarify the researcher's thinking and served as guidelines for the planning and conduct of the teaching/learning experiment. They were also useful to the nurse teachers in the different colleges who carried out the teaching of the control and experimental groups of students. They provided information to the students as to what was to be learned and what was expected of them. In addition, by prescribing specific outcomes, they facilitated the assessment of the students' progress.

Because objectives are an efficient method of communication of intent, it was considered important to withhold information about certain of them from the participants in the early stages of the experiment. The cognitive and affective objectives related to the course of instruction were known to students and staff before the course began, and provided the guidelines for the teaching, learning and the end-of-course assessment. All other objectives were disclosed only after the experiment was complete, lest they influence participants' opinions and therefore their evaluation of the experiment.

Three levels of objectives

Goodwin & Klausmeier (1975) differentiate between objectives in education in terms of their degree of generality or of specificity. They state that first level objectives are of high generality and low specificity — such objectives are formulated at national level, with the purposes of providing objectives for local educational agencies to consider. A parallel in nursing is the GNC (Scotland), the national body that provides the syllabus and general guidelines for the colleges of nursing to follow in compiling their own programmes for education and training. At level 2, Goodwin & Klausmeier consider the degrees of generality and of specificity to be moderate. This is the level concerned with implicit instructional objectives formulated at local level with the purpose of suggesting objectives for classroom teachers to consider. There is a parallel here with certain of the objectives which were formulated for the experiment in regard to factors in the integration problem. Such factors could be considered neither wholly general nor wholly specific, as they will operate to a certain extent in many, though not all, of the colleges of nursing. The objectives on this second level are objectives numbers 1 to 11(B), in the list on pages 75 and 76.

The third level in Goodwin & Klausmeier's classification was that of low generality but high specificity. These were the explicit instructional objectives familiar to most teachers acquainted with the writings of Benjamin Bloom (1956) and R. F. Mager (1962). Such objectives are normally formulated at classroom level, by the teacher or occasionally nowadays by both teacher and students (Boydell, 1976).

Objectives 11 (c), (d), 12 and 13 were level 3, i.e. of high specificity, and were closely related to the entirely course-specific cognitive learning objectives shown in Appendix A. The latter were expressed in the more generally accepted format for end-of-course objectives, i.e. they were behaviourally stated, readily measurable objectives. In addition to the cognitive objectives, there were also affective objectives (see again Appendix A) concerned with students' attitudes, values and feelings about nursing care as a result of their exposure to the experimental course. Although the cognitive objectives were unequivocally at level 3 in Goodwin & Klausmeier's trilogy, the affective objectives of this experiment dealt with ways of thinking and acting and therefore with a process which was potentially generalisable to other teaching/learning situations and other nursing situations. They were thus capable of contributing to the general aim of the research at a slightly higher level than were the knowledge objectives.

THE RESEARCH APPROACH — ILLUMINATIVE EVALUATION

The Gestalt concept, that the whole is more than the sum of the constituent parts was basic to the approach adopted in this research. A study which has as its aim the facilitation of integration of theory and practice in nursing cannot but involve four distinct groups of people, student nurses, nurse teachers, ward staff and patients, and two separate environments, i.e. service and education, or hospital and college, each with their own particular ethos.

The appropriate techniques for evaluation of such a complex scene were deemed to be those of illuminative evaluation. Parlett & Hamilton (1972) state:

> Illuminative evaluation is not a standard methodological package but a general research strategy (which) aims to be both adaptable and eclectic. The choice of research tactics follows not from research doctrine, but from decisions in each case as to the best available techniques. (p. 15)

Over the last decade the emphasis in educational research has tended to move away from the 'clean and tidy', strictly controlled setting of the psychological laboratory, using what has been termed the 'agricultural-botany' paradigm, and into the much more 'untidy' world of the reality of the educational scene (Tuckman, 1978). That reality tends to be even more untidy if it includes, as it does in nursing education, the world of work. With the change in emphasis came the 'alternative' paradigm which made use of ethnographic techniques, developed by anthropologists and community-study sociologists. Wilson (1977) describes the rationale underlying the ethnographic methodology as based on two sets of hypotheses about human behaviour:

a. the naturalistic-ecological hypothesis that human behaviour is significantly influenced by the settings in which it occurs, from which it follows that it is essential to study events in their natural settings, and

b. the qualitative-phenomenological hypothesis that human behaviour often has more meaning than its observable 'facts'.

From this it follows that the researcher can only understand human behaviour insofar as he has an understanding of the framework within which the subjects interpret their thoughts, feelings and actions. Taken to its extreme, this particular approach could become as unwieldy and as unrealistic in the furtherance of educational research as its predecessor, the strictly controlled pure research of the traditional approach. Where the latter stressed objectivity, measurement and proven facts, the former, in the endeavour to gain a wider understanding, required prior knowledge of the setting and/or close observation of it by the researcher, and thus introduced many problems of subjectivity of interpretation. However, with the realisation of this threat to any subsequent generalisation of research findings resulting from the approach, came the development of a considerable number of different techniques of design, data gathering and data analysis.

Illuminative evaluation, by taking account of the wider contexts within which educational programmes function, has been placed within the alternative paradigm. It is by definition a more eclectic approach in which no one particular research method or technique is paramount. The problem is said to define the method used, and such an approach seemed particularly apposite to this research. Just as the design of the educational experiment had to be such that it was sufficiently flexible to fit into the different college of nursing adaptations of the nurse education and training programme, so the evaluation techniques had to be adaptable and capable of use in the different settings.

The aims of illuminative evaluation are to study the innovatory programme, and were in this case applied to the experiment in teaching and learning to nurse. Parlett & Hamilton (1972) state these aims as follows:

> to study . . . how it operates; how it is influenced by the various school situations in which it is applied; what those directly concerned regard as its advantages and disadvantages; and how students' intellectual tasks and academic experience are most affected. It aims to discover and document what it is like to be participating in the scheme, whether as teacher or pupil. (p. 9)

ILLUMINATIVE EVALUATION APPLIED

Translated into the situation in nurse education, and in this research, this approach required that account be taken of aspects of the physical, organisational and educational milieux of college and hospital, and of the pre-experiment opinions of student nurses, college staff, i.e. the officially designated teachers in nursing, and ward trained staff — ward sisters, staff nurses and enrolled nurses. It required documentation and description of the day to day conduct of the experiment which was organised by the researcher in a form of participant observation. Following the experiment, traditional outcome measures such as test scores were not ignored, but the focal point was the evaluation of the aim and objectives of the experimental teaching/learning method, and opinions of the involved staff (both teachers and ward staff) and students about the advantages and disadvantages of the innovation as they saw it, i.e. what it was like to be participating in it.

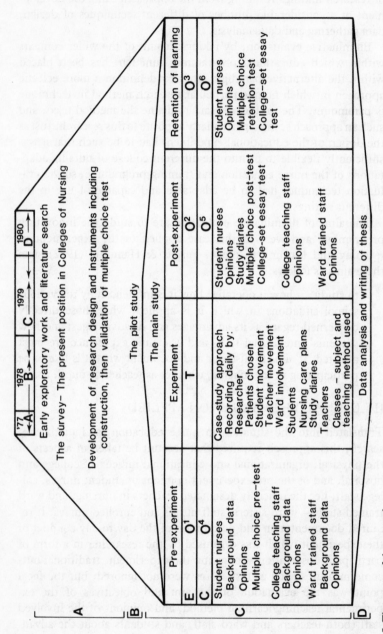

Fig. 5 The stages of the research

	Pre-experiment	Experiment	Post-experiment	Retention of learning
E	O¹	T	O²	O³
C	O⁴		O⁵	O⁶
C	Student nurses Background data Opinions Multiple choice pre-test College teaching staff Background data Opinions Ward trained staff Background data Opinions	Case-study approach Recording daily by: Researcher Patients chosen Student movement Teacher movement Ward involvement Students Nursing care plans Study diaries Teachers Classes – subject and teaching method used	Student nurses Opinions Study diaries Multiple choice post-test College-set essay test College teaching staff Opinions Ward trained staff Opinions	Student nurses Opinions Multiple choice retention test College-set essay test

A — Early exploratory work and literature search
B — The survey – The present position in Colleges of Nursing
C — Development of research design and instruments including construction, then validation of multiple choice test
  The pilot study
  The main study
D — Data analysis and writing of thesis

'77 → A → 1978 → B → C → 1979 → D → 1980 →

Figure 5 outlines the stages of the research.

Simultaneously with the gradual evolvement of the design of the research and the experiment, a survey of a number of colleges of nursing was carried out, which yielded descriptive background data relevant to the system of nurse education. This supplemented and updated the researcher's own knowledge of the system. Prior to the pilot and main studies, various research tools were designed and pre-piloted. These included questionnaires and a 100-item multiple-choice test of knowledge of the subject matter of the course. The latter was validated prior to its use in the pilot and main studies. Following the pilot study in one college of nursing and its associated hospital, the main study was conducted in five colleges of nursing in Scotland.

The design incorporated features associated with both the traditional and the alternative paradigms. Reference to Figure 6 will show the use of what Campbell & Stanley (1966) refer to as a 'true experimental design . . . the pretest-posttest control group design' (p. 13). This was the part of the research in which traditional methods were used in order to attain a measure of control over certain relevant variables. Quantitative data were obtained in the form of test scores from the students, which, although recognised as not entirely objective data, made possible the calculation of learning gains for the students in the control and experimental groups. The subjective assessment by all the participants completed the evaluation of the experiment.

No hypotheses

The reader familiar with experimental research may well at this point be searching for the statement of hypotheses.

Entwistle (1973) stated:

> as far as educational research is concerned, the paradigm of the hypothetico-deductive method is an ideal rarely achieved. The complexity of (students') behaviour in the classroom often leaves research workers still at the stage of hypothesis hunting. Elaborate theories with accurate prediction lie in the future. (p. 18).

As this research took place not only within the classroom, but also within the wards, hypotheses were not used in the evaluation of the experiment for the following reasons: (a) hypotheses imply an objectivity and a cause-and-effect relationship which was not wholly justifiable, either in this research or in most educational research; (b) very many extraneous variables, for example related to the students' cognitive strategies and the different patients who helped provide the nursing care content of the course, would have intervened between the independent variable, i.e. the teaching/learning method, and the dependent variables, i.e. the opinions of the participants and the test scores of the students; and (c) hypotheses tend to place the emphasis upon the readily quantifiable, in this case the test scores, and, although these were a necessary part of the outcome measurements in this research, they were not paramount. The scores were but one small part of the whole, and it was the whole which was the concern of this evaluation.

6

Details of the design and the experiment

DESIGN OF THE EXPERIMENT

The design chosen for this experiment is one considered by Campbell & Stanley (1966), and many others (Pilliner, 1973; Burroughs, 1975), as the best available for educational research which takes place, not in the controlled, artificial setting of the laboratory, but in the real world of the classroom. The latter type of educational research, Pilliner states, is likely to convey more conviction and have maximum relevance to the needs of both teacher and student, but it entails problems related to the control of extraneous variables, or interfering influences which can tend to obscure or confound the effects which are of particular interest. Such influences Campbell & Stanley refer to as threats to the validity of the experiment, both the internal validity, in that the research results can be accepted as being a function of the experimental treatment, rather than of other uncontrolled variables; and the external validity, which affects the question of generalisability of the results. Among the factors which these authors consider jeopardise internal validity are (1) history, events other than the experimental treatment occurring between a pre- and post-experiment measure, (2) maturation, processes within the subjects operating simply as a function of the passage of time, e.g. growing more tired, growing hungrier as coffee-time approaches, (3) testing, the effects of taking a test upon the scores of a subsequent testing, (4) instrumentation, changes in scorers or scoring, (5) statistical regression, occurring where groups have been selected on the basis of extreme scores, (6) selection bias and (7) experimental mortality, i.e. differential loss of respondents from the comparison groups. External validity or generalisability of results may be threatened by the possibility that the pre-testing may alter subjects' responsiveness to the experimental situation, i.e. that the results may be those of groups 'warmed up by the pre-test' (Campbell & Stanley, 1966) and therefore not generalisable to an unpretested population. There is also the problem of any interaction effects from selection bias and the experimental treatment, and the threat of the well-known 'Hawthorne effect' (Roethlisberger & Dickson, 1939), i.e. the reactive effects of the experiment *per se.*

Bearing all of this in mind, the design which was decided upon for this experiment was the pre-test/post-test control group design — what is termed a true experimental design, as shown in Figure 6. The above design was adapted in this study in two ways. Firstly, a retention of learning observation or measurement was added. This was made when the subjects next returned to Block, a period of some three to six months after observations 2 and 4 (Fig. 6). Secondly, the experiment was replicated on four occasions, following its first use in the pilot study, and later use in the first of the main study colleges.

The adapted design used in this research is shown in Figure 7. The two groups employed were the experimental group who received the treatment, and the control group who did not receive the treatment.

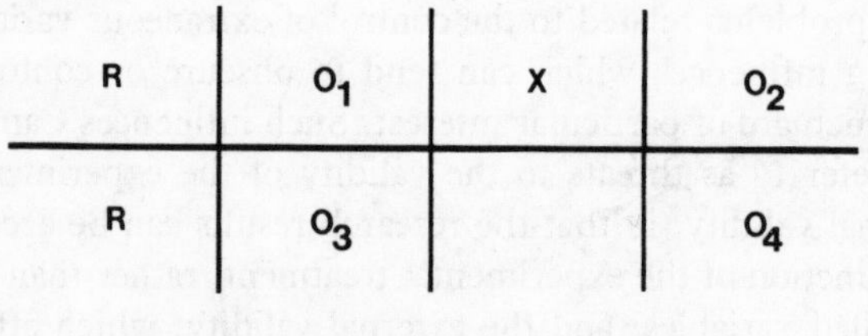

R	O_1	X	O_2
R	O_3		O_4

R indicates groups chosen by randomisation
O indicates an observation or measurement
X indicates a treatment or independent variable

Fig. 6 Pre-test/Post-test control group design (Campbell and Stanley, 1966, p. 13)

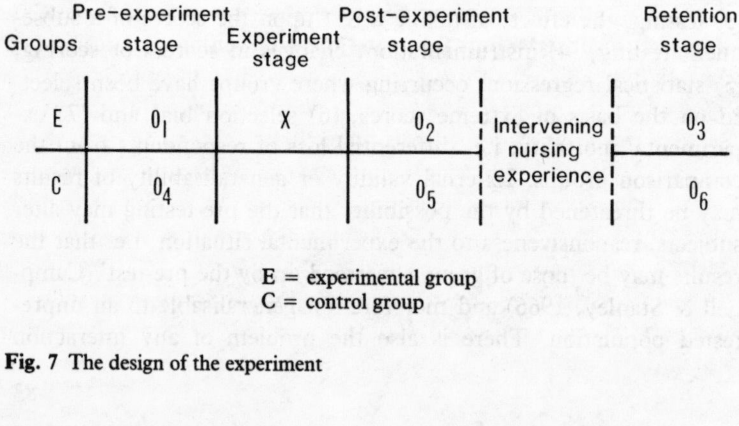

Groups	Pre-experiment stage	Experiment stage	Post-experiment stage		Retention stage
E	O_1	X	O_2	Intervening nursing experience	O_3
C	O_4		O_5		O_6

E = experimental group
C = control group

Fig. 7 The design of the experiment

It is perhaps misleading to depict the comparison between the groups in the above design as between 'X' or 'no X'. Campbell & Stanley point to the over-simplification of the position which is suggested in the diagrammatic representation. In the case of this nursing education experiment, the control group students were taught the same course content as the experimental group students. It was the experience of the integrated college teaching and ward practice of related nursing which represented the 'X', the absence of that experience which represented the 'no X'.

A critical feature of the experiment design was the allocation of subjects to experimental and control groups by a process of randomisation, which was preceded by matching the subjects on a variable considered relevant — in this case knowledge of the subject matter of the course and of related but more general nursing. Burroughs (1975) stated:

> There is a single correct procedure for matching. (Students) are matched on such variables as are selected. Then each matched pair is taken and one of the (students) allocated *at random* to one group and the other (student) to the other group. The matching comes first and the grouping comes second rather than the other way round. (p. 64)

This was exactly the procedure adopted in this experiment. The difficulty of controlling the variable of prior relevant experience and knowledge was overcome by the administration of the pre-test, i.e. the specifically designed and validated multiple-choice test (0_1 and 0_4 in Figure 7) which tested that knowledge, and yielded scores on which subjects were 'paired' or matched. Details of the randomisation procedure, and of the construction and validation of the test are given in the original thesis.

The experiment design controlled for all the sources of internal invalidity although it was recognised that, by the addition of the third set of observations following the intervening practical experience, the factor of history may have been less well controlled. However, to counteract this, testing of both groups was always carried out simultaneously. Most importantly, the long intervening period, of varied experience, between the treatment and observations 3 and 6, constituted a serious threat to the validity of the final stage of the experiment. Experimental mortality was also very slightly increased due to the passage of time.

The use of the pre-test, which was one limit to generalisability of the results, was considered justified, and indeed very important in this experiment, simply because of the problem in nurse education, of controlling the amount and type of practical experience and ward teaching each student nurse receives — quite apart from the use she may make of such opportunity. The limitation to generalisation posed by the pre-test was mitigated by the fact that testing is a regular feature in nurse education, and also by the fact that no one of the students, at the time of pre-testing, knew of the experiment which was to follow for some of them, therefore none was aware of the significance of the test.

The problem of selection bias was dealt with as far as possible, by the use of the replicate sample design. In all, six colleges of nursing participated, one in the pilot and five in the main study, and there was no reason to suppose that these colleges were unrepresentative of the colleges of nursing in Scotland.

The independent variable or 'treatment'

The independent variable was, in essence, a method of teaching nursing. A planned teaching/learning unit of concurrent theory and practice of nursing took place within the normal theoretical component of the basic general nurse education and training programme. During the hours allocated to the nursing lectures for one subject in their curriculum, students in the experimental group spent part of their time in the wards, under the supervision of their teachers from college, giving total nursing care to patients who had been chosen because their conditions related directly to the subject matter of the course. For the remaining hours, these students returned to the college, to participate with the same teachers, in a seminar or tutorial in which they discussed the nursing care they had been giving, relating it to their patients' needs and to the relevant textbooks and lecture material.

The independent variable was therefore a college and ward-based method of teaching/learning, but it also included three factors which were inseparable from the intervention and must be considered a part of the treatment. These were the introduction and use of a handout in the form of a 'nursing care plan' note-taking framework, with accompanying instructions, a development which in fact arose as a result of the pilot study; the accent upon the concept of individualised patient care; and the use of the patient, rather than the task assignment pattern of organisation of nursing work.

With the exception of one college in which the experimental group constituted an entire class, the experimental method was experienced by only a part of each class of student nurses, i.e. each class was divided into control and experimental groups. For the identical number of hours that the latter group experienced the altered method of teaching nursing, the control group received teaching based upon the same content, and utilising the same cognitive objectives, but entirely college-based. All the teaching was carried out by the teachers of the college concerned, and those teaching the experimental group did not teach that particular subject to the control group, nor did the opposite occur, i.e. control group teachers did not teach nursing to the experimental group. Students were in separate classrooms for this subject. However, any other course content, for example medical staff lectures, films or visits to appropriate departments, was shared by students in both groups. The essential difference between the control and experimental groups can be seen in Figure 8.

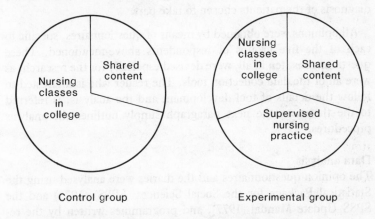

Fig. 8 Essential difference between control and experimental groups

The dependent variables
The dependent variables were:

(1) the opinions of the students of the experimental group, their teachers and the ward staff involved, about the experimental teaching method, and also in regard to the achievement or otherwise of the objectives of the experiment;

(2) the opinions of the students of the control group and their teachers as a result of their experience of the experiment; and

(3) the scores from the students on the objective tests and the essays.

Other data collected
Other data which were collected, as they were considered relevant

to the general description of the context within which the experiment took place, were:

(1) opinions of students, college teaching staff and ward staff as to certain aspects of the nurse education and training programme. These opinions were again obtained by means of specifically designed questionnaires;

(2) information about student nurse study patterns — obtained by means of a daily study diary kept by each student during the course of the experiment;

(3) records of classes given and teaching methods used by teachers of both control and experimental groups; and

(4) records of experimental group student and teacher movement throughout the various wards during the experiment, and of the diagnosis of the patients chosen to take part.

All opinions were obtained by means of questionnaires, specific to each of the five groups of respondents above-mentioned. These questionnaires, ten in all, were devised especially for the research, as were all of the data collection tools. The reader who is interested to follow the details of tool development and the analysis, is referred to the thesis, as the next paragraph simply outlines the analysis procedures.

Data analysis
The opinion questionnaires and the diaries were analysed using the Statistical Package for the Social Sciences (SPSS) (1975) and the SPSS Update Manual (1977), and programmes written by the researcher. Apart from the calculation of a Kendall Coefficient of Concordance (Siegel, 1956) with regard to student teaching method preference, statistics were not used in the analysis of the questionnaire or diary data, as they were not considered relevant. Scores on the multiple choice test were calculated by a short programme added to the Rasch Item Analysis Model (Wright & Mead, 1977) which had been used for the item analysis when the test was constructed and validated. Scores on the essays were obtained by the issue of the scripts to three neutral markers, all of whom were General Nursing Council for Scotland examiners, and, in the case of the post-essays, also to the teachers of the college concerned. Statistics were used in the analysis of the test and essay scores. Measurement of central tendency, and of dispersion, Pearson product-moment correlations, sign test, t-test and analysis of variance were carried out using the Statistical Package for the Social Sciences (1975). Significance testing was deemed appropriate as gener-

alisation of the results to the population from which the sample was drawn, is possible, albeit to a limited extent.

Analysis took place across colleges, with the exception of the test results from the College where the entire class had composed the experimental group. When between college differences were relevant, these were reported, as were any within college differences, although the latter were less frequently found.

THE SAMPLE

The student nurses

The population, from which the sample was drawn, was student nurses currently undertaking the General Nursing Council (Scotland) course of education and training leading to registration on the General Register, by means of the traditional college of nursing and hospital-based programme.

A total of 119 students were involved, which number represents 3.8% of the total number of student nurses in training in 1978. (General Nursing Council (Scotland) 1978). They were all in that part of the theoretical component of their programme which included the subject matter of the experiment. *Only* those students, the large majority of the sample, who were encountering that subject matter for the first time were eligible for inclusion in the control and experimental groups in so far as all outcome measurements were concerned. A very few students, who were either previously trained, previously enrolled, were re-sitting part of their course, or were graduates of a non-nursing degree programme were members of some classes. These students had studied material relevant to the subject matter of the experiment previously, so, although they were in one sense a part of the control group, they contributed to the outcome measurements only in the opinion questionnaires and diaries.

The students of College III were an exception to the above. These students were undertaking an experimental comprehensive programme of training and were in their pre-registration period. They were therefore at a later stage of training (two and a half years), and they were included in order to measure the effect of the experiment in these different circumstances.

Selection of a particular class of students was dependent upon the researcher's choice of college, and the presence of these students in the appropriate Block in that college at a time which was suitable to the researcher's timetable.

The colleges

The pilot study college was chosen following a survey interview there, when the Director and her staff expressed an immediate interest in 'trying out' the experiment which had been explained during the course of the interview.

The main study colleges, of which there were five, represented 26% of the total of 19 colleges of nursing and midwifery in Scotland. Utilising information from the Directory of Schools of Nursing (DHSS, 1977) it was possible to carefully select these to be as representative as possible of these 19 colleges. Two were large colleges, attached to teaching hospitals in the major cities, two were much smaller in size, and situated, one in a county town and the other in a rural area, and one was of medium size, and conducted the experimental comprehensive programme. It was situated in a moderately sized coastal town. The selection of the colleges was governed by their accessibility from Edinburgh, the researcher's base — the furthest was fifty miles distant from this; and by the presence in each college, at a time suitable to the researcher's timetable, of a Block in which the subject matter of the experiment was taught. Selection was also dependent upon the willingness to participate of the staff of the college. There was one college in which this participation was not forthcoming.

The teachers

All were on the staff of the colleges. Altogether 72 teachers, 14% of all teachers in post in Scotland in 1978, completed pre-experiment questionnaires. A total of 19 teachers were involved in the experiment, 11 in teaching the experimental group students and 8 with the control group students. This number represents 3.7% of the teachers in Scotland.

In each college, the initial choice by the researcher of a suitable Block in terms of (a) appropriate course content, and (b) the timing vis-à-vis the research timetable, dictated which teachers would be approached and asked if they were willing to take part in the actual experiment. As each college operated the 'Salmon-type' team system of formal organisation, then those teachers who were approached were members of the team responsible for the chosen Block. In only one college was it necessary to request one additional teacher from another 'team', and this was also the only college in which it was possible to allocate teachers to the control or experimental group teaching by randomisation.

Teachers of both control and experimental groups were from RNT and RCT grades, and in so far as the teaching of the subject matter of the experiment was concerned, i.e. medical/surgical nursing of patients with disease of the gastrointestinal system, no teacher taught both groups; control group teachers remained with the control group for that particular subject each day, and experimental group teachers remained with the experimental group. It was quite likely that at another time of the day, and for another subject, teachers would be involved in teaching the entire class.

The hospitals
The hospitals which provided the practical experience for the experimental group students were those which normally did so for the colleges in the study. There were seven in all because, in two of the colleges, it was the practice to utilise two different hospitals in order to obtain the requisite practical experience for their students.

The ward staff
Trained staff of general medical and surgical wards in the seven hospitals in which the main study experiment took place completed pre-experiment questionnaires, a total of 224. It was not possible to ascertain what proportion of medical and surgical ward trained staff this figure represented.

There were 58 ward sisters, staff nurses and enrolled nurses of general medical and surgical wards directly involved in the experiment. Their selection was a result of their having in their ward, at the time of the experiment, patients whose diagnosis and condition made them suitable for inclusion in the numbers of those to whom the experimental group students gave care, and also was dependent upon them being the nurse in charge of the ward on a day when the experimental group students and their teachers were at work therein. The total of 58 included staff from the pilot study college, the only situation in which pilot study data was included in the main analysis.

The patients
In all 110 patients were given care by the experimental group students, and thus they were also participants in the experiment. Patients were chosen, following consultations between the researcher and the ward staff, when their diagnosis and condition were considered suitable for the experimental group students' needs in terms of learning experience. The question of patient consent was a matter of considerable concern and this is dealt with on page 106, as is the question of evaluation by the patients of the care they received from the experimental group students.

THE TASK

The task (Tuckman, 1978) was described as the 'vehicle for introducing treatments' as it was neither an independent nor a dependent variable. The task or activity in which all students in the study participated was the learning of the content, or the subject matter of the course, i.e. the nursing care of patients with gastrointestinal disease, as outlined in the current General Nursing Council (Scotland) Syllabus, previously referred to.

The task in the context of the Block timetable

Within the framework of the above-mentioned Syllabus, each individual college of nursing was free to make its own interpretation. Essential to the acceptance and implementation of the experiment was that the researcher be aware of these individual differences and that the design of the experimental method be sufficiently flexible to take account of these differences, without any loss of control over the integration of theory and practice, the direct link between what was being taught in the college and what was being practised in the wards by the experimental group students.

A typical Block day (Fig. 9) contains five or six periods, each of from 45 minutes to one hour in length, during which students receive teaching on a variety of subjects, from nurse teachers, and visiting lecturers, including, for example, medical staff, the pharmacist, microbiologist, chaplain, psychologist, physiotherapist, and representatives from social and voluntary services. In some colleges, a week, or a number of consecutive days will be devoted to one predominant theme or subject, but it is a more common practice to adopt a more eclectic approach and to timetable two, three

Days	Periods						
	1	C	2	3	L	4	5
Monday							
Tuesday							
Wednesday							
Thursday							
Friday							

Fig. 9 Typical block day/week (includes several subjects)
1 — 5 = Class Periods
C = Coffee Break
L = Lunch Break

or more quite different subjects during the course of a week. Medical staff lectures, where they were included, tended to be preceded or followed by related biology and nursing lectures, given by the nurse teachers.

The organisation of the timetable is the responsibility of a nurse teacher, either a senior tutor or the teacher in charge of the student group, and the teaching methods employed are normally entirely at the discretion of each individual lecturer.

THE EXPERIMENT IN THE CONTEXT OF THE BLOCK

The way in which the experiment fitted in to the system of timetabling is shown in Figures 10 and 11.

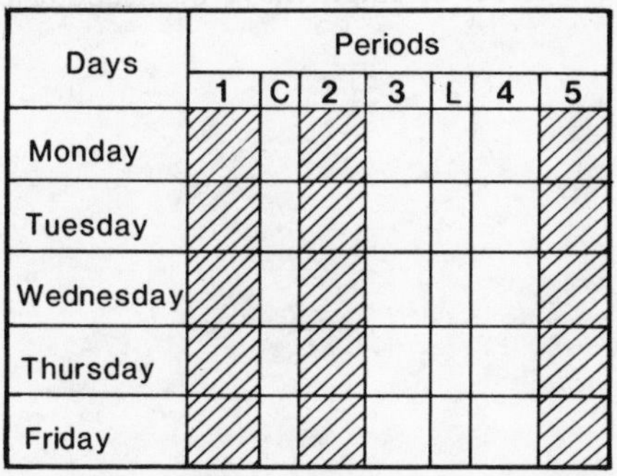

Days	Periods						
	1	C	2	3	L	4	5
Monday							
Tuesday							
Wednesday							
Thursday							
Friday							

Fig. 10 Control group day/week during experiment
Hatched area = Nursing care of patients with gastrointestinal disease.
Clear area = normal Block Programme — mixture of subjects — all students together.

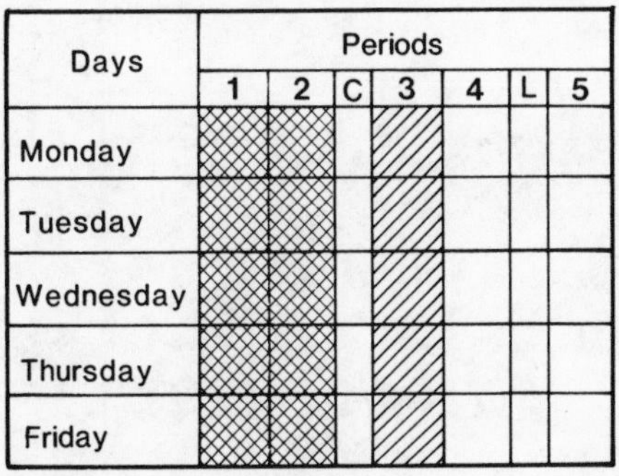

Days	Periods						
	1	2	C	3	4	L	5
Monday							
Tuesday							
Wednesday							
Thursday							
Friday							

Fig. 11 Experimental group day/week during experiment —
Hatched and clear areas as above.
Cross-hatched area where student was on supervised ward practice.

For the control group students, the teaching of gastrointestinal nursing occupied the first two periods and the last period of the day, and for the experimental group students, this teaching took place during the first three periods of the day — the first two in the wards, and the third, in the college. The experimental group began and finished their day earlier than the control group, for reasons which were in part ward-related, and in part due to concern for the control group, in that it was considered more acceptable on educational grounds, to break the control group students' experience of the subject matter, as three consecutive periods of gastrointestinal nursing might have proved somewhat 'indigestible'!

For the remaining periods of the Block day, students from both groups shared whatever content was organised in their timetable. This might have included medical staff lectures on diseases of the gastrointestinal system, or might have been about another subject altogether.

7

The process of implementation

This chapter describes the organisation of the experiment. The procedures are detailed for each of the four stages, i.e. the pre-experiment, experiment, post-experiment and retention stages. In all except the retention stage, three separate groups of nursing personnel were involved — the teachers or college staff, the ward sisters and staff nurses or hospital staff, and the student nurses. At each stage, information was both given to, and received from members of all three groups — a process of communication, negotiation and explanation on the one hand and a process of data collection on the other. Inclusion of a college depended not only upon the consent of the college and later of the hospital staff and of the students, but also upon the occurrence of an appropriate Block in college at a time which fitted to the researcher's timetable. If the college had been included in the earlier survey, data were already available in regard to the timing of Blocks. If the college had been selected by the researcher following her perusal of the Directory of Schools of Nursing (DHSS, 1977), then information as to the Blocks was obtained at an initial interview with the Director.

THE PILOT STUDY

A pilot study was carried out in the summer of 1978, in a large college of nursing and its associated teaching hospital. The purpose of the pilot study was to provide the possibility for a complete trial run of the experiment in all its stages, to allow the administration of the various newly constructed data collection instruments, and to give the researcher experience in attempting the subsequent analysis of the data.

The college chosen, the training programme, and the students in the pilot sample were all representative of those it was intended to include in the main study.

The experience of the pilot study proved invaluable. It permitted the logistics of the experiment to be worked through as a result of which a number of small but important modifications were made. The experience gained during the pilot study made it an indispensable preparation for the main study.

THE MAIN STUDY

Pre-experiment procedures
The first contact, in each college, was with the Director of Nurse Education, and this was followed by meetings between the researcher, the Director and her teaching staff. Subsequently the researcher met with the Divisional Nursing Officer of the hospital, and her administrative and ward staff, and finally the student nurses who were to be directly involved in the research were contacted.

Meeting with teachers of the control and experimental groups
As soon as it could be arranged, following the initial meeting with the Director, at which permission had been granted to go ahead with the experiment, the researcher met with the teachers responsible for the Block in which the experiment was to be carried out. At this meeting the details of the experiment and what it would involve for the teachers were explained, any questions they raised were discussed and the researcher then formally asked whether the teachers were prepared to participate* — an essential question as it was the college teachers who did the teaching, not the researcher. Thereafter, consent achieved, the teachers and the researcher discussed carefully the basic organisational framework into which the experiment would be fitted in the unique milieu of each college.

Essential points which required consideration and action at this preliminary stage of the planning are discussed below.

Timetabling details

Dates of the course. The proposed dates for the gastrointestinal system nursing lectures, and where these were placed in relation to medical staff lectures were ascertained. Was it possible for the nursing content to follow closely upon the medical staff lectures, and to ensure both were complete by the end of the experiment? In some cases this was easily arranged, in others some alterations were made in order to achieve the desired dates and ordering of subject matter.

Hours and course content. The number of hours and the course con-

---

* There was one college in which neither teachers nor students were given this choice, on the express instruction of the Director of Nurse Education.

tent were examined to ensure that a *minimum* of twelve hours were devoted to the teaching of nursing. This figure would permit of at least four mornings spent on the wards, an arbitrary minimum decided on by the researcher as constituting a viable experiment time. In the event only one college had that minimum of 12 hours — the time allocated to the nursing content of the subject matter ranged from 12 to 24 hours in the various colleges.

The ward experience took place on consecutive mornings — where any impediments to this had been already planned into the timetable, e.g. visiting lecturers, previously arranged Department visits, these were resited. The placing of the requisite hours, in the timetable, was finalised and it was ensured that none other than gastrointestinal nursing lectures occupied the last hour of the afternoon for the control group on the days when the experimental group students were in the wards. Thus the latter group could start and finish their day one hour ahead of the control group students (see Figs. 9 to 11 on pp. 92 and 93). The exact time of the morning start for the experimental group students and their teachers was also decided at this point, and was related to the normal starting time of the day duty shift on the wards. However, there was sufficient flexibility in the arrangement so that, should the ward sisters subsequently wish to delay the arrival of the students and their teachers on the wards by 15 minutes, this would be possible. It was ensured that two separate classrooms were available to the two groups whenever these were required, i.e. when gastrointestinal nursing was to be taught.

Insertion of research-required hours. Insertion of research-required time, at the appropriate positions in the timetable, was also done at this stage. In all, six sessions were necessary. The pre-test required one hour, and had to be completed before any of the relevant lecture material was given, preferably immediately before such material, or with as short a time interval as possible. The pre-experiment opinion questionnaire was inserted prior to any explanation by the researcher to the students about the experiment and the linking of theory and practice in their nursing education. Half an hour was allocated to this, and a further half hour was required subsequently for a full explanation of the experiment to the students, and the intimation to them of their random allocation to control and experimental groups. The day prior to the experiment, the first of the divided classes was scheduled. This was a one hour period of preparation in which both groups, separately, would receive an introduction to the subject matter of the course. The experimental group teachers and their students would use the nursing care plans, the guide thereto, and the learning objectives for the first time at this session, and final arrangements for the next morning on the wards would be made. The control group teachers and students would also use these same learning objectives for the first time during their own session. A one hour period for the post-test had to be fitted in to the timetable. This was always scheduled to follow the college-set essay test, and, whenever possible, was sited in the period immediately after the essay. The college-set essay, although an integral part of the evaluation of the research experiment was not considered to be a 'research-required hour' as it was a normal part of the Block programme in all colleges. Finally, and occupying only 15 minutes on the last day of the experiment, usually after both tests had been completed, a short period was set aside for the students in both groups to complete the post-experiment questionnaires.

The student numbers
The number of students in the class who were undertaking the subject matter for the first time as part of their basic RGN training, and thus were eligible for inclusion in control or experimental groups, was ascertained. The total number of eligible students decided the number of randomised pairs, and influenced the decision, by the researcher and the teachers, as to the size of the experimental group. The ratio of students to teacher, while on supervised ward practice had been decided upon previously, by the researcher, and was one teacher to four students. Thus each experimental group was composed of multiples of four.

The teacher numbers
The minimum number of teachers required was dependent upon the size of the experimental group, with its ratio of one teacher to four students, and an additional, and equal number, to share the teaching of the control group.

Availability of practical experience
The number of general medical and general surgical beds, and wards, was ascertained — this gave some indication of the numbers of suitable patients likely to be available to the experimental group students. The proximity of such general medical and surgical experience was checked. In order not to cause disruption to college timetabling for either group of students, it was necessary that experimental group students should require no more than 15 minutes to return to college from the supervised ward practice.

Learning objectives presented
Finally, at this first meeting of the researcher and the teachers who were to be directly involved in the experiment, the learning objectives were presented and discussed. The views of the teachers as to the suitability of the objectives for use with both control and experimental groups were obtained and in all cases were favourable.

Meeting with all of the college teachers

Following discussion of and agreement on all the above matters the next step was to meet with all of the college teaching staff together, with the primary aim of informing them of the research experiment. Opportunity was given for questions and discussion, as the details of the research were explained. The teachers were informed that the Divisional Nursing Officer would be contacted, but that the students should not be consulted, until permission to go ahead had been received from the hospital staff.

At this meeting all staff were informed that questionnaires would be issued to them by the researcher when she returned to begin the experiment. In these questionnaires they would be asked to give their opinions on matters related to nurse education and training, but it was stressed that their response was not obligatory.

Introduction of experimental group teachers to the experimental teaching methods

All subsequent meetings in the college were those between the researcher and the experimental group teachers, and were devoted to the preparation of the teachers for the experiment and the teaching methods it involved. Following the first of such meetings, which was in the nature of a workshop, any further sessions were arranged only if desired by the teachers. The learning objectives, nursing care plans and the guide thereto were given to the teachers at the first preparatory meeting in each college, and these, together with the undernoted recommendations of the researcher in regard to the conduct of the experiment and the teaching approach, were worked through.

1. Once the students, and their teachers, had received the report from the ward staff about their patient(s), the teacher should spend a short time with the students, so that together they could decide what were the priorities for each morning, which patients should be cared for first, whether students required special supervision or demonstration of any care they had been requested by the ward staff to carry out. This should all be planned before students and

teachers introduced themselves to their patients, in order to allow the morning to run smoothly for all the students and especially for the patients.

2. Students were likely to require help and guidance as to what to observe in the practical setting, and also to make the link between their theoretical teaching and their work with the patients. The stress should be on specific theory in relation to gastrointestinal nursing care, although previously learned theory in relation to basic care should be included.

3. As essential part of the experiment was that students should also have time, and guidance, in making notes and extracting relevant material from the Kardex and the patient's case notes.

4. The discussion time, during the seminar following the period of ward practice each morning, should be used to encourage students to relate theory and practice in regard to their own patient and his care. This could be best achieved if teachers worked with the students they had supervised that morning, guiding them to make the appropriate integrating observations, which process could be facilitated by the students' completion of their nursing care plans.

5. The researcher would endeavour to find for each day, patients with similar conditions, although perhaps at different stages of their illness. By so doing, it was hoped to enable students to appreciate that the same 'label' in terms of diagnosis, did not necessarily mean the same treatment or nursing care. They should be enouraged to compare their own patient's care with those of their classmates, and so come to a knowledge of the principles of nursing care in patients with gastrointestinal conditions.

6. The aim should be to have students see patients as individuals, to give them individualised care, in relation to their needs, and to see that as compatible with any type of ward organisation. Students should be encouraged to view their patient as a person with a life outside the hospital and his present illness, to take time to talk with him, to use any extra time to communicate more with him.

7. Students should be encouraged to ask questions.

8. Part of each day's seminar should be devoted to teaching of relevant subject matter which was not available in direct relationship to patient care on that day, and teachers were advised to plan such sessions, together with deciding which of them should teach. The ratio of one to four should be unnecessary for such, possibly more formal teaching.

9. Finally, as it had transpired that teachers were, for the most

part, unfamiliar with nursing care plans, and a little unsure of the teaching approach although unanimously in approval of it, the researcher suggested that, prior to a second meeting, the experimental group teachers should each work through a nursing care plan, in relation to an imaginary patient, and this could then be discussed, and any difficulties or questions dealt with.

Thus was the all important matter of the experimental teaching method introduced to those who were to use it. Although the researcher intended to influence the *approach* to the teaching, the fact that the college teachers carried out all the teaching without further supervision, or the presence of the researcher in the experimental group classroom, did mean that there was no effective control over that important variable. It is contended that in the real world of the classroom it is not possible to control teaching and the human teacher.

Meetings with the hospital nursing staff
Negotiations with the hospital nursing staff began with a meeting between the researcher and the Divisional Nursing Officer of the hospital, or hospitals, concerned with the provision of the appropriate practical experience for the students. At this meeting the experiment was fully explained and the Divisional Nursing Officer and/or in some cases, the Senior Nursing Officer asked whether she was prepared to have her hospital participate in the research. The fact that the college were prepared to take part was known to the Divisional Nursing Officer, but the researcher stressed that the participation of the hospital, although crucial to the experiment, was not a foregone conclusion. Following this preliminary meeting, which in each case had a successful outcome, the researcher prepared an information sheet giving the details of the experiment as it would affect the ward staff, and this sheet was used as the basis of information-giving and discussion at the next meeting with hospital staff. This was arranged by the Divisional or Senior Nursing Officer, and was between the researcher and the ward sisters or charge nurses of the general medical and surgical wards. All the wards which normally provided general medical and surgical experience for the students were represented at that meeting, if not by the nurse in charge, then by her deputy. Unit Nursing Officers for these wards were either informed or present. The information sheet was handed out to everyone at the commencement of the meeting, so that as the researcher explained what would be involved in their participation in the experiment, the staff could fol-

low each step, and ask questions if they wished. Information about the number of students likely to come to the wards, their stage of training, exactly when they would come on duty and when they would leave, and exactly what they would do when there, was given. The procedure for the choice of patients was explained, as was the matter of who would take responsibility for the patient while the Block nurse was caring for him, and also who would be responsible for the supervision of the student. The ward staff retained the information sheet, so that they could refer to it as necessary, and also so that the sisters could go over the information with their ward staff.

On two occasions, the Divisional Nursing Officer offered to approach the ward staff and explain the experiment, but the researcher considered it most important that she personally explain the research and the experiment to the ward staff, for three reasons: (1) to try to ensure no alteration of the information, which to some extent is inevitable when a message is given by an intermediary, (2) to obtain face to face contact from the outset with the staff with whom the researcher would work during the experiment, and (3) to present as clearly as possible, the opportunity for any ward sister to decline to participate. Although it was accepted that there would be considerable pressure to participate, as all ward sisters knew the senior nursing service staff had agreed to the study, it was felt there would be more freedom for dissent, or doubtful acceptance, if the 'unknown' researcher were to put the question. In all but one hospital, the researcher was alone with the ward staff. In the other, the senior and unit nursing officers were present.

In two hospitals, suggestions were made by the Divisional Nursing Officer that potentially 'difficult' wards might not be used for the experiment. However, it was considered important not to avoid such areas, and it was explained that research done only where attitudes were considered to be receptive would be of little practical use to the profession. Thus, at no time, was any general medical or surgical ward omitted from the study if it contained patients who were suitable for inclusion, and for providing nursing care for the experimental group students.

At the close of the meeting the researcher explained, in the same way as with the college teachers, about the questionnaires.

Meetings with the student nurses
On three occasions before the experiment began, the researcher met the whole class of students who were to take part in the research.

At the first meeting, the researcher introduced herself with a very brief description of her background in nursing and the information that she was currently engaged in research into nurse education. This meeting took place immediately prior to the first medical staff lecture on the subject matter of the course, and was for the purpose of the administration of the objective test. The test was handed out to the students, with the explanation that it was a part of the research project, and a request for the co-operation of the students in completing it. They were informed that the test had nothing at all to do with their college, and that their marks would not be divulged to their teachers, nor put into their records, but were solely for the purpose of the research. Students were asked to complete the frontispiece details, and then to read the second page, which contained the sample test items and the explanation of completion details. Anything which they did not understand at that point was clarified. Students were then asked to work steadily through the test, assured that they were not expected to know all of the answers at this stage of their training, and asked to try to resist the temptation to make an outright guess at any answers. They were told to leave blank those questions to which they really did not know the answer and, if corrections were made, to make them very clearly. The time allowed for test completion was 55 minutes. The test was collected as it was completed by the students and later that same day, the frontispiece was detached and retained. The remaining sheets were identified with the correct student number and the answers transferred to the computer programme aforementioned as expeditiously as possible, as it was on these scores that the random allocation of students to control and experimental groups took place.

The purpose of the next meeting was to ask the students to fill in the pre-experiment questionnaire, for which half an hour was available, and which was used to the full by most of the student respondents. The researcher explained that the questionnaire sought their *opinions* about their education as a nurse, that there were no right or wrong answers, but it was important to the research, and to the profession, to know what the students thought. Specific instructions were given that they should try to answer every question. It was pointed out that in a few questions, two alternative responses were all that were given. In such cases, they should try to choose the response which came closest to their opinion. Although their name was asked for at the head of the questionnaire, it was explained that this was necessary so that a code number could be inserted, but that at no time would any individual student and her answers ever be identified. All replies would remain confidential, a matter for which the researcher would be responsible. In each college, the researcher was alone with the students, and it was made clear to the students that participation was not obligatory. However, far from reluctance, their response was unanimously one of interest and willingness to complete the questionnaires.

The last meeting in which the whole class met together with the researcher before the experiment took place was the occasion when the experiment was fully explained. The identical information sheet which had been prepared for the ward staff was given to all the students. They retained this, and it served as a focus for the discussion. The fact that there would be the two groups, of experimental and control students was discussed and explained, although the details of how the allocation had been done was not divulged until the post-experiment meeting with the students. As carefully as possible, the researcher made it clear to the students that they could decide to opt out of direct participation in the research if they so wished, although in fact they would remain in class with the control group students, as would other class members not eligible for inclusion because of their previous experience of the course material. It was also explained that it was necessary to obtain the students' consent to participation before the announcement of allocation to control or experimental groups was made, in the interests of the validity of any results from the experiment. (Only two students did opt out, and they were from the pilot study college.)

On the weekday prior to the start of the experiment, the researcher met the experimental group students, with their teachers, and in the first ten minutes of the class, gave out the nursing care plans, guides thereto, the learning objectives, and the diaries and discussed their use briefly. Arrangements about a rendezvous point for the first morning of the experiment were made, together with information about patient allocation, if this was available at that point. Students worked in pairs, the same pair together throughout the ward practice, making the decision about their co-workers themselves. Dependent upon the amount of care required by the various patients, students might share one patient during a morning session, or have one patient each, helping each other as and when necessary in the giving of the morning care. The question of supply of sufficient of the above-mentioned forms, and where they would be most suitably kept throughout the experiment, was also dealt with, and the researcher then left the students and their teachers to commence their first class on the subject matter of the experiment.

The researcher then joined the control group class and their teacher, and explained about the shared learning objectives, and the supply, completion and collection of the control group diaries.

The selection of the patients

As had been agreed previously with the ward staff, on the day prior
to the experiment, whether a weekday or a Sunday, the researcher
visited all the medical and surgical wards of the hospital, and using
the Kardex and case notes, listed all suitable patients. This list,
with brief comments, was then checked with the ward sister or staff
nurse on duty, and any special circumstances which would contra-
indicate the allocation of any patient to the students in the experimental group were noted. When this task was completed, the
researcher contacted the experimental group teachers, and together
they made the choice of patients who would receive care the next
morning. Finally, the researcher returned to the wards to leave a
brightly coloured card on the Kardex, which stated which pa-
tient(s) the classroom nurses would care for the following morning.
In most cases, the teachers also visited the wards, to consult the
case notes and the Kardex. It was not routine to meet the patient at
this time, nor to inform him that he would be given care by two
classroom nurses on the following morning, a matter which is discussed on page 106.

The task of obtaining this initial information about the patients
occupied from less than one hour in one hospital, to a maximum
time of five hours in the largest hospital in the study. Throughout
the course of the experiment, it was never again necessary to make
a formal list of suitable patients; this information was updated regularly and informally, as the teachers and the researcher met with
the ward staff and patients day by day.

Issue and collection of the pre-experiment questionnaires

A list of all college staff was obtained from the college office, and
from the hospital senior nursing officers a list of the ward sisters
and staff nurses of the general medical and surgical wards. This latter information was often given in the form of photocopied off-duty
lists, which proved a very helpful method for the researcher and a
very simple and speedy method for the service staff providing the
information. All questionnaires were issued with a covering letter
and delivered by the researcher as she toured the hospital on the
day prior to the experiment, collecting information about the patients. They were left at the Nurses' Station for those staff not on
duty when the researcher visited the ward. Completed questionnaires were collected from the Nurses' Station, or directly from the
respondents again when the researcher was in the wards each day.
College staff questionnaires were handed to staff on the first day of
the experiment, and were either collected later by the researcher, or
were left on her desk by respondents. The presence of the research-

er on the wards and in the college, together with the fact that, when in a ward, she generally asked if there were any questionnaires ready for collection, no doubt contributed to what was a high response rate.

Accommodation for the researcher

In each college, accommodation was required, and made available to the researcher. A number of the papers connected with the research required safe-keeping, and in some cases the researcher had a personal office, in others, a desk which could be locked.

PROCEDURES DURING THE EXPERIMENT

The questions of patient permission and evaluation of care, also confidentiality of information.

In a few instances, usually when a chosen patient was alert, reasonably fit and had noticed and shown an interest in the fact that the researcher, or the experimental group students and their teachers were in the ward, he or she was approached, the proposed plan for his care the next morning explained, and his permission and co-operation requested. In most cases, however, prior explanation was not given and permission was not sought. There were two reasons for this. Firstly, ward staff considered that patients rarely, if ever, knew who would come to give them their morning care the next day, and were unaccustomed to having any choice in the matter. Secondly, as a result of experience during the pilot study, when patients had been informed prior to the event, and their permission requested, it was discovered that, for some, this was an anxiety-provoking experience. However carefully the explanation was given, by the researcher or the ward staff, a few patients, having had the night to think it over, had come to the conclusion that there was something seriously wrong for them to have been singled out in this way. It was therefore decided to abandon the routine of informing the patient, and requesting permission. As it transpired, the fact that the experimental group students were with their patient(s) for one to two hours ensured that the patients became aware that they had been chosen and why, which fact then became much more a matter of interest, and for some patients a matter of pride, rather than of anxiety.

The researcher met, and talked with every patient, some time after they had received care from the experimental group students, and always an attempt was made to obtain the patient's evaluation of the care given. Again, during the pilot study this had been attempted in a somewhat structured way. Shields (1978) and Hale (1974), both from the other side of the Atlantic, wrote of their work in obtaining patient opinion of the nursing care they had received. Hale devised a 'patient satisfaction scale' on which degrees of satisfaction with nursing care received could be assessed on a five point scale ranging from highly satisfied to dissatisfied. A very much simplified version of this scale was used during the first days of the pilot study, in an attempt to encourage patients to evaluate the care they had received, but this proved very foreign to them, somewhat embarrassing, and was abandoned as most unlikely to yield valid results.

The researcher, and the students with their teachers, were privy to much confidential information about their patients, and were also making notes which were taken out from the ward. Students were cautioned about this matter, and no patients' names appeared on their care plans. In addition, students were asked to ensure their care plans did not lie unattended by the patient's bedside, or elsewhere in the ward or college. The researcher did have names, diagnoses and ward numbers on her form listing the available patients, and this was kept very carefully.

Day-to-day organisation
Each day, the researcher added to the list of available patients, conferred with ward staff and with the teachers and students of the experimental group, and finalised the choice of patients for the next day. She then ensured that ward staff knew exactly who the experimental group students would take care of the next day, removed any out-of-date coloured card from the Kardex and replaced it with a current version, if applicable. Each day, also, the researcher visited patients who had been given care by the experimental group students, and spoke with them.

Daily record keeping by the researcher included a careful note of each student's experience, in terms of the diagnosis and condition of the patients to whom she had given care. As this information accumulated for the individual students in the experimental group, careful attention was paid to the types of learning experience being provided. The researcher and the teachers endeavoured to choose as balanced, and as wide a range of relevant practice as was possible for each student.

Teacher and student movement throughout the different wards was also recorded daily, as was the ward usage throughout the experiment. At the end of each day, and before experimental group students left college, they knew who their patient was for the next day, which ward he was in, which teacher was their supervisor and where they should meet the next morning.

Student nurses in both groups completed study diaries and these were collected daily by the researcher. This provided a valuable daily contact with the control group students. Stocks of diaries, and of nursing care plans and continuation sheets for the experimental group students were replenished daily.

Teachers daily completed their record of classes given, but this information was not collected by the researcher until the completion of the experiment. Finally, on the researcher's regular ward and college visits, questionnaires were collected and checked off on the list.

POST-EXPERIMENT PROCEDURES

Post-experiment questionnaires were issued to ward trained staff, to teachers of the experimental and control groups, and to students in both groups. Care was taken to ensure that *only* those ward staff who had been in charge of the ward on days when the experimental group students were giving nursing care there, received these questionnaires. The off-duty sheets aforementioned proved most useful. If a ward sister or staff nurse was to be off duty on the last days of the experiment, her questionnaire was handed out before she left for days off. In a very few cases, it was necessary to provide a stamped addressed envelope for the return of the questionnaire, but otherwise these were collected by the same methods as were employed with the pre-experiment questionnaires.

For both control and experimental group students, the college-set essay and the multiple choice test were taken, if not on the day the experiment ended, then on the first working day thereafter. Instructions for the former were given at the head of the test paper, and were little different from normal practice in the various colleges. There were only two specific instructions to the students (a) that they should not put names on the papers, but use their research number, which was handed out to each student at the start of the session, and (b) that they should use black ink pens for the script, and if they preferred it, pencil for any diagrams. It was explained that the papers would be photocopied, hence the necessity to use the black ink pens with which they had been provided by the researcher. The objective (multiple choice) test was presented to the students without prior warning. They did not know that they were to take the identical test for a second time, as it was thought that foreknowledge of that event might have led to deliberate attempts by the students to recall question items after the first administration of the test, thus distorting subsequent results.

Instructions and timing of the test were similar to those of the first administration, as was the method of marking. The essay scripts were photocopied, and one set of scripts sent, by post, to each of the three neutral markers, together with a covering letter and a copy of the test paper from which the name of the college had been removed. The original scripts were then returned to the college, as the post-essay was marked also by the college teachers, and it was their mark which was used in the college records. The scripts were normally returned to the college on the day following the examination, to ensure that as little time as possible was lost between the taking of the essay test and the marking and issue of results to the students.

The last task the students carried out at the close of the experiment was the completion of their post-experiment questionnaires, and again these were introduced in a similar manner to previously, in that students were asked to be frank in their expression of their opinions, informed that there was no right or wrong reply to any question, and assured of confidentiality.

In each college, an informal session was arranged with the control and experimental groups before the researcher left, at which students were free to ply the researcher with questions and engage in discussion on all aspects of the research.

Finally, an arrangement was made with the teachers for a mutually convenient date for the last stage of the experiment, the retention of learning assessment. This return was not intimated to the students at this point.

RETENTION STAGE PROCEDURES

The final stage of the experiment normally took place when the class of students was next in college or Block. Shortly before this previously arranged return date, negotiations recommenced with the teachers, in order to finalise times and the classroom venue. On two occasions, some class members were undertaking practical experience on the required afternoon, and their recall to the college was arranged by the teachers, in co-operation with their service colleagues. All students therefore became aware, shortly prior to the event, that they were to meet with the researcher again, but were not told of the reason. This was most important, in order to ensure that they did not study for the tests. The differential preparation which might have resulted from prior knowledge of the testing session would have constituted a very important interfering variable.

On meeting with the students, the researcher announced the programme for the afternoon, said that it would occupy approximately two hours, that it was positively the last stage of the research in which they would have an active role to play, and requested their co-operation. In this introductory talk, it was explained that the two tests taken at the end of the experiment were to be re-taken, in identical form. The essay was to be written first, followed by the objective test, and then, for the experimental group students only, the short follow-up questionnaire was to be completed. In order to reduce the anticipated, and natural anxiety of the students, they were reassured that it was a normal process for people to forget a certain amount of what had been learned, asked to try not to worry about how much they felt they might have forgotten, and to work steadily through the two tests. These were timed as before, and again black pens were issued and used. Research numbers only appeared on the essays. Names did appear on the slightly amended frontispiece for the objective test, which was required in order to obtain important information about each students' intervening practical experience, betwixt post-experiment and retention stages. The process for correction of scripts and objective tests was as before with one exception. College teachers were not involved in the marking of their students' scripts. Students were told of this prior to taking the tests, again in the interests of reducing possible anxieties.

At the close of this, the final part of the research, all students were given the opportunity of receiving their results from all the tests they had taken. They were told this would be done, if they wished, by means of a personal letter sent to them by the researcher. Students were then reassured that there was no more testing to be done, and that the researcher hoped to return, but this time to report, and discuss with them, the results of the research.

SUMMARY — THE MAIN STUDY IN SYNOPSIS

The main study was conducted in five colleges of nursing and their associated hospitals. Its timespan, from the first negotiation with the Director of Nurse Education of College I until the retention stage in College V is shown in Figure 12, and was from 20th July 1978 until 22nd October 1979, a period of 16 months.

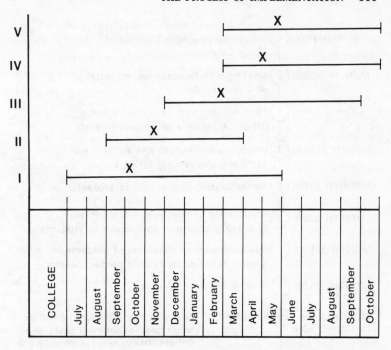

Key: Line denotes time from first negotiation with Director of Nurse Education to date of retention stage in each college. X = position of experiment in each college

Fig. 12 Timespan of main study and date of experiment in each of the five colleges of nursing

Although the research followed the procedures described in this chapter in all colleges, each had their individual learning milieux and thus the process of implementation was not identical in each college. An example of the way in which the experiment ran its course is shown in the Figures 13 to 17 and Tables 1–3. This particular college required less experimental group teacher preparation than any other in the main study, and the control group teachers made use of a wider variety of teaching methods than did any of their colleagues in other colleges. However, to extract an example in order to outline the process of implementation in tabular form, may prove helpful to those readers who prefer Figures and Tables to text. The implementation of the experiment in each college is outlined in this way in the thesis.

MONTH 1/7th ① Initial interview with Director of
Nurse Education

MONTH 1/28th ② Meeting with Director and directly
involved teachers

MONTH 2/9th ③ First meeting with Divisional Nursing
Officer. Meeting with all college staff

MONTH 2/20th ④ Meeting with medical and surgical ward
staff and unit nursing officers

MONTH 3/6th ⑤ Administration of pre-test to students

MONTH 3/9th ⑥ Preparation of teachers. Administration
of pre-experiment questionnaire to students

MONTH 3/13th ⑦ Announcement of allocation of students to
groups, followed by first of divided classes

MONTH 3/15th ⑧ Initial selection of patients

MONTH 3/ 16th to 23rd +⑨+ EXPERIMENT (includes day after ward practice
when post-experiment tests and
questionnaires were administered)

MONTH 9/11th ⑩ Retention of learning assessment and follow
up questionnaire

Fig. 13 College: synopsis of implementation, progress and conclusion of
experiment

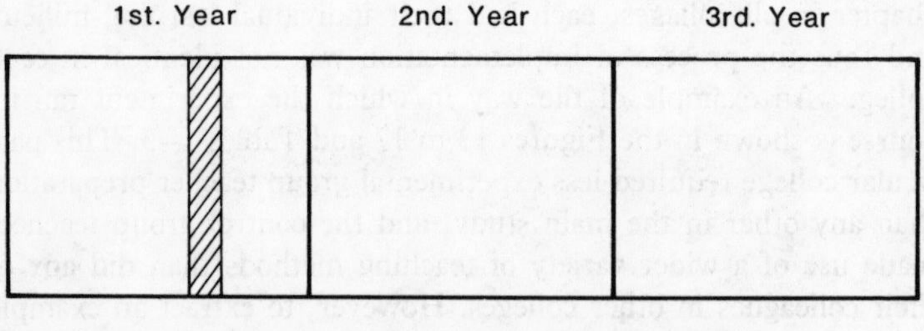

1st. Year   2nd. Year   3rd. Year

Fig. 14 College: position of experiment in students' training programme

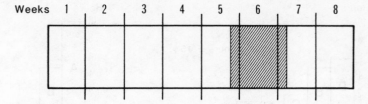

Fig. 15 College: position of experiment in Block programme

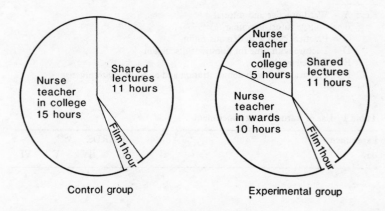

Fig. 16 College: control and experimental group experience of course content. Care of patients with gastrointestinal disease

Total Hours on Subject — 27

Shared lectures (medical staff) — spread over 10 days occupied 11 hours = 41% of course

Shared film — occupied 1 hour = 4% of course

Nursing lectures (nurse teachers) — spread over 5 days occupied 15 hours = 55% of course

Experimental group — 10 hours in ward practice — 37% } 55%
5 hours in college teaching — 18%

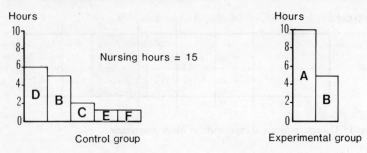

Fig. 17 College: teaching methods used for nursing content. Control and experimental groups

Key: A = Ward practice and tutorial
     B = College tutorial/seminar
     C = Practical class with demonstration
     D = Lecture with time for questions/discussion
     E = Guided study
     F = Practical class with demonstration and opportunity to practise

Table 1 Use of wards during experiment

Experiment day	WARDS					
	I	II	III	IV	V	VI
1	★	★		★		★
2		★★	★★			
3	★		★	★	★	
4	★		★	★	★	
5		★	★★★			
No. of student hours per ward	12	16	28	12	8	4

Key to wards: Wards I to III — Surgical
              IV to VI — Medical

Table 2 Movement of students through wards

Experiment day	Student pairs			
	A	B	C	D
1	VI	IV	I	II
2	II	II	III	III
3	V	IV	III	I
4	I	III	IV	V
5	III	III	II	III
No. of different wards per pair during experiment	5	3	4	4

Table 3   Movement of teachers through wards with student pairs

Experiment day	Teacher X		Teacher Y		No. of wards per experiment day
	In ward	With pair	In ward	With pair	
1	I & II	C & D	VI & IV	A & B	4
2	III	C & D	II	A & B	2
3	I & III	C & D	IV & V	A & B	4
4	I & III	A & B	IV & V	C & D	4
5	III	A & B	II & III	C & D	2
Total no. of wards and student pairs	3	4	5	4	

Note: 1 teacher taught only in surgical wards
       1 teacher taught in both medical and surgical wards

The research findings

In accordance with the aims of illuminative evaluation, which are to study the innovation in the setting in which it operates, Chapters 8 to 11 (PART 3A) report the opinions of the student nurses, ward trained staff and teachers about some aspects of the teaching/learning milieu in general nursing, as they see it. Part 3B, Chapters 12 to 16, reports the views of the same three groups about the experimental teaching/learning method, i.e. in Parlett & Hamilton's terms, what it was like to participate in it, and also describes the results of the tests and essays, and the students' study patterns.

This is, in the main, qualitative data, the subjective assessment of the world of work and education prior to, and during the experiment. There are some who would dismiss qualitative data as 'not real research', but it is contended that it is our thoughts and feelings about our work which have a profound influence on what we do — thus, it seems very important to endeavour to find out what nurses think and feel about their work, and about any innovation.

The following abbreviations are used throughout Part 3:
EN   — Enrolled Nurse
SN   — Staff Nurse
RNT(SNT) — Registered Nurse Teacher/Tutor
RCT(CT)   — Registered Clinical Teacher
WS   — Ward Sister or Charge Nurse

The research findings

The teaching/learning milieu
prior to the experiment

8

Characteristics of the samples

The students

The composition of the sample of 119 student nurses who completed the pre-experiment opinion questionnaire is shown in Table 4. Of the sample 88% were undertaking RGN training as a first and basic experience of nursing, and 12% had either a previous training or previous experience of the course material by some other means. A majority of the students had practical experience of only 16 weeks equally divided between general medical and general surgical wards. The remainder of the sample had more, both in time and variety.

The response rate was 100%.

Table 4 Pre-experiment: students. Composition of student sample by college

Student nurses	I	Colleges II	III	IV		N = 119 (100%)
Basic RGN	27	9	27	23	19	105 (88%)
Pre-trained	-	-	2	-	-	2 (1.7%)
Previously enrolled	-	1	1	2	-	4 (3.3%)
Previous experience of course material	-	-	-	6	2	8 (7%)
Total from each college	27	10	30	31	21	119 (100%)
	23%	8%	25%	26%	18%	100%

The ward trained staff

The ward sister and staff nurse opinion questionnaire was issued to all trained staff working in the general medical and surgical wards of the hospitals which provided the practical experience for students from the five colleges of nursing. Each hospital was identified by the same Roman numeral as its associated college, e.g. Hospital I is the hospital for College I. For Colleges I and III respectively, two hospitals were available and normally utilised to provide the general medical and surgical experience for the experimental group students, hence the A and B in these cases in Table 5.

Table 5 shows the distribution of the three grades of trained staff in the sample, and Figure 18 indicates the length of time in their present grade of the ward sisters and staff nurses. There were six male nurses, i.e. five charge nurses and one staff nurse, in the sample.

Table 5 Pre-experiment: ward trained staff.
Distribution of sample by staff grade and hospital

Hospital		Ward sisters	Staff nurses	Enrolled nurses	Total N	%
I	A	19	73	-	92	(41)
	B	1	7	-	8	(4)
II		9	13	-	22	(10)
III	A	4	11	7	22	(10)
	B	2	5	5	12	(5)
IV		18	24	1	43	(19)
V		14	11	-	25	(11)
Totals in each grade		67	144	13	224	(100%)
		30%	64%	6%	100%	

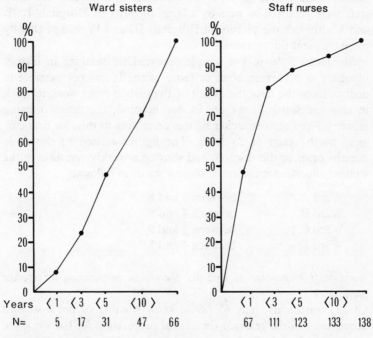

Fig. 18 Pre-experiment: ward trained staff. Cumulative percentages of numbers of trained staff and length of time in present grade

There was a very different composition of these two main grades of staff in the sample, in terms of time-span in their present grade. Of the 66 ward sisters, 53% had been in that grade for five years or longer, compared with only 11% of the 138 staff nurses, of whom almost half (49%) had been staff nurses for less than one year.

A total of 31 medical wards and 25 surgical wards were represented by the 224 staff, 109 (49%) of whom worked in medical wards and 115 (51%) on surgical wards.

The response rate was as follows:

Hospital I	93%
Hospital II	100%
Hospital III	92%
Hospital IV	96%
Hospital V	93%

Ratios of staff to learners and stability of staff and student numbers
Reported ratios of staff to learners (i.e. both student and pupil nurses) for these medical and surgical wards were not lower than 1 : 2 and in a majority of both medical and surgical wards these ratios ranged from 1 : 1.5 to 1 : 1. Fluctuations in numbers of trained staff were reported as rare by a large majority in Hospitals I, II, and V although the picture in Hospitals III and IV was of slightly more frequent fluctuations.

Altogether 93% of the sample reported fluctuations in learner numbers as occurring often or fairly often. It was not possible to deduce from the data the extent of fluctuation from week to week in any one ward. However, in one hospital, the senior nursing officer offered the researcher figures pertaining to this, for four surgical wards, each of 23 beds. The figures related to the three months prior to the research and showed a weekly variation in the student allocation numbers to these 4 wards as follows:

Ward A	between 3 and 8
Ward B	between 4 and 9
Ward C	between 5 and 9
Ward D	between 4 and 8

Ward staff knowledge of students' theoretical preparation for specific ward work
Of 223 ward staff, only 65 (29%) knew whether or not a student nurse had had the relevant theoretical preparation for the work she was required to do in their particular ward. 70% of the sample acknowledged that they did not know. These respondents were from

all three grades. There was no evidence of a relationship between knowledge of student preparation and length of time in grade of the respondents.

The teachers*

Table 6 shows the distribution of the 72 teachers who completed the pre-experiment opinion questionnaires throughout the five colleges. The questionnaires were not identical for the registered nurse teacher and for the registered clinical teacher.

Table 6   Pre-experiment: teachers.
Distribution of grades throughout colleges

| College | Registered Nurse Teachers | | | |
	SNT	RNT	RCT	Total N = (100%)
I	2	13	10	25	(35%)
II	1	3	2	6	(8%)
III	4	6	12**	22	(31%)
IV	2	4*	2	8	(11%)
V	2	5	4	11	(15%)
Totals	11	31*	30**	72	(100%)
		42			
% of each grade		58%	42%		(100%)

* includes one unregistered teacher
** includes one unregistered clinical teacher

The response rate ranged from 100% in three colleges, to 89% and 80% respectively in the others.

The teachers' length of experience in post, and as ward sisters or charge nurses is shown in Figures 19 to 22, in relation to both grades of teacher.

Deployment of teachers

In all five colleges staff worked in 'teams', headed by a senior tutor; each team responsible for several student intakes throughout their training period. With the exception of College II, the smallest college in the study, where staff in the two teams intermingled and tended to share the workload, there were, in effect, a number of virtually autonomous small colleges within each college.

---

* Where the full title of each of the two grades of nurse teacher, i.e. the Registered Nurse Teacher (which includes SNT and RNT) and the Registered Clinical Teacher (RCT) is not given, the RNT is referred to as the tutor, and the RCT as the clinical teacher. Where both grades are referred to, the term teacher is used.

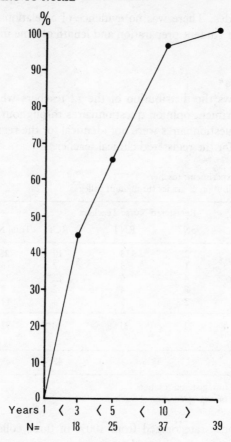

Fig. 19 Pre-experiment: teachers. Cumulative percentage — registered nurse teacher — length of time in present grade

The most common method of arriving at an individual teacher's teaching commitment was to have discussion within her team, under the leadership of the senior tutor. However, four of the eleven senior tutors said their own teaching commitment was self-allocated, and in the smallest college, teaching commitment was decided by discussion with all college staff.

For the clinical teachers, all but one of whom taught in wards, and most of whom taught in both wards and college, the day to day commitment of ward teaching was left to their own discretion, though clearly influenced by the exigencies of the hospital, the wards and the number of learners on duty at the times when the clinical teacher was available. They were peripatetic — none worked

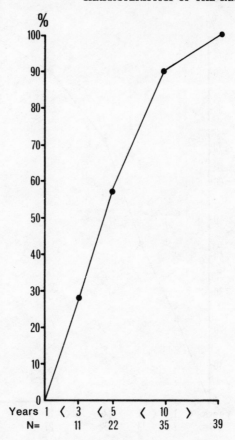

Fig. 20 Pre-experiment: teachers. Cumulative percentage — registered nurse teacher — length of time as ward sister/charge nurse

in only one ward or unit. One did, however, work in all operating theatres, and this person was outstanding as the one teacher whose role resembled, to some extent, that of the clinical nurse specialist. She taught only the subject of her 'specialty', i.e. theatre nursing and theatre technique, and this to students in the basic RGN programme only, although auxiliaries and Operating Department Attendants joined in her tutorials at times. In addition, she was responsible for a very small amount of college teaching, again of her 'specialty' subject.

In contrast, not only did all but seven of the 42 tutors have a responsibility to teach in a number of different training programmes, and in some cases, in post-basic courses too, but all taught *most* of

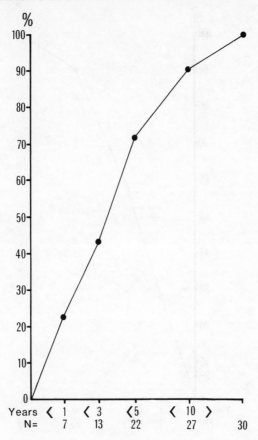

Fig. 21 Pre-experiment: teachers. Cumulative percentage — registered clinical teacher — length of time in present grade

the subjects in the General Nursing Council (Scotland) syllabus for any programmes with which they were involved. For the 31 tutors who considered they had 'specialist' knowledge of some nursing subject, 29 (93%) of them also taught that subject, but usually only to students within their own team's responsibility. Only one tutor mentioned teaching her specialty within other teams. Two comments about specialty teaching were as follows:

There are some areas which I used to consider my specialty, but there has been some erosion by the need to teach most things.

Continual teaching of one subject is economical of time and

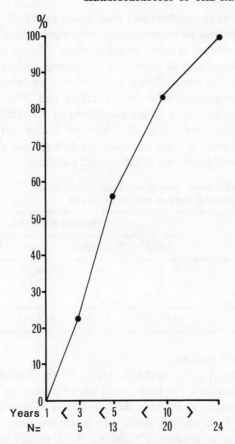

Fig. 22 Pre-experiment: teachers. Cumulative percentage — registered clinical teacher — length of time as ward sister/charge nurse

can be of more value to the students... The longer you are away from running the ward, the more difficult it is to keep up to date with your specialty, particularly regarding new drugs and treatments.

With regard to teaching in the wards, only three tutors considered they often taught there, although a further 28 included some ward teaching in their work remit.

In addition to their teaching commitment, 28 tutors, including the 11 senior tutors, had overall administrative responsibility for student intakes throughout all of their training period, and 32 tutors acted as personal tutor to learners, ranging in number from 14 to 82, and in the case of one senior tutor — 150.

Meeting between teachers and ward trained staff

All tutors felt they had some contact with ward trained staff — 80% considering this to be often or fairly often. Clinical teachers were not asked about this, as they were considered, rightly or wrongly, to be daily in the wards. There was, however, evidence of complete lack of communication between teachers and 37% of the ward trained staff, and of a larger proportion of the staff nurses and enrolled nurses (see Table 7). The staff nurses were the group contributing most to ward teaching, yet 45% of their number never met or consulted with any of the trained teachers.

Table 7   Pre-experiment: ward trained staff.
Frequency of meetings with education staff

Staff grade	Frequency of meeting				
	Often	Fairly often	Rarely	Never	N=
Ward sister	4	13	36	13	66
Staff nurse	3	17	59	64	143
Enrolled nurse	3	1	4	5	13
All grades N =	10(4%)	31(14%)	99(45%)	82(37%)	222(100%)

Purpose of such meetings

The majority of such meetings related to the assessment and/or teaching of learners. For many ward staff, this was the only contact with the teachers, which begs the question as to how much contact there might be if learners spent very much less time on the wards than they do at present. Of the 63 ward staff who mentioned teaching and/or assessment of learners, 31 said this contact was only with the clinical teacher.

> When the clinical teacher comes to teach. (*EN* — Enrolled Nurse)
> Contact is with the clinical teacher who spends one week in three on the ward teaching students. No contact is made with any other college staff. (*EN*)

Assessment was related to the progress of students and for the most part appeared to be somewhat informal. It took place mainly with clinical teachers. There was evidence, from one college, however, that efforts were being made by college staff to visit learners during each ward experience, if possible about half way through their allocated time there — so-called 'interim visits' — in order to assess progress.

Fairly often with clinical teachers, rarely with tutors, except for interim visits. (*WS* — Ward Sister or Charge Nurse)
Interim visits about midway through each learner's experience in that ward . . . I also meet night staff at fairly regular intervals. (*RNT* — Registered Nurse Tutor)

Less formal assessment of progress, e.g.:

The clinical teacher comes to the wards and asks how the student is coping, then has a chat with the student or watches her carry out a procedure. (*WS*)

There was evidence, in many responses, of visits triggered off by 'problems' or difficulties, e.g.:

Usually to discuss poor performance or difficulties encountered by student/pupil nurse. (*WS*)

or

Only if there is a 'bad' student nurse. (*WS*)

Meetings between education and service staff also took place for the purpose of up-dating knowledge. There was evidence that the clinical teacher, especially, was seen as a resource person:

I often consult with the clinical teacher, as she can advise as to what the student is allowed to do in the ward, and is up-to-date in new methods, and can offer valuable advice. (*EN*)

Tutors spoke of the necessity to consult ward staff to up-date lectures, to exchange information, e.g.:

To keep up-to-date with changing techniques. (*RNT*)
Contact with ward nursing staff to find out about new treatments, investigations and also drugs currently used. Also to see new equipment being used. (*RNT*)

A very few comments looked towards the importance of communication for service/education relations, e.g.:

To build up good relationships, so I am welcome.
To keep track of new things. (*RNT*)
To maintain a continuity between self and service staff. (*RNT*)

The dependence of teachers upon ward staff to 'permit' them to work with patients was inherent in the following 'purposes of contact' given by ward staff:

To ask permission to work with students. (*SN* — Staff Nurse)
The form is usually a short discussion in sister's office. The
purpose is to see if it is convenient to carry out teaching at a
specific time in the ward. (*SN*)
To be asked for a student to be released for a tutorial or for
teaching nursing care. (*SN*)

It is interesting that no teacher mentioned 'asking permission'.

In only two hospitals did respondents mention formal meetings
between education and service staff — in one, these meetings did
not include staff nurses, only ward sisters. In the other, the Procedure Committee was the venue of joint co-operation.

There was no evidence of meetings or contacts initiated by the
ward staff apart from the seeking of information from the clinical
teacher when she was present in the ward, i.e. education had come
to service in the first instance.

9

Classroom teaching and learning

METHODS OF TEACHING/LEARNING PREFERRED BY STUDENT NURSES

Students were asked to rank eight methods of teaching/learning in order of preference, giving the rank '1' for the method best liked, to '8' for the method least liked. The students' rankings were then pooled across all five colleges, and a mean rank obtained for each method. The resulting preference profile is shown in Figure 23 together with the key to the listed methods.

Kendall's coefficient of concordance statistical test (Siegel, 1956) was applied to the student rankings, and the Kendall W of .41 which was obtained, reflected a degree of agreement among the students ranking the 8 methods which was significantly more than would have occurred by chance ($p < .001$).

Clearly placed as the 'best liked method' was the ward tutorial, and this method retained first place in the students' preferences when these were inspected for each individual college. Equally clear was the students' dislike of self-directed study. Over all five colleges, and for four of the five individual colleges, this was the 'least liked method'. Sixth, seventh and eighth ranks, i.e. the least popular methods over all five colleges and in each individual college, were ascribed to guided study, straight lectures and self-directed study. In all colleges, where practical classes were concerned, there was a slight preference for those which gave opportunity for the student not simply to listen and observe, but also to practise.

Participation in class discussions

Student nurses were asked about their frequency of participation, when the opportunity was given to ask questions or have discussion in class.

More than half the respondents, i.e. 66 (56%) considered they rarely or never participated and 52 (44%) that they participated often or fairly often. Results from Colleges I, II and III showed

131

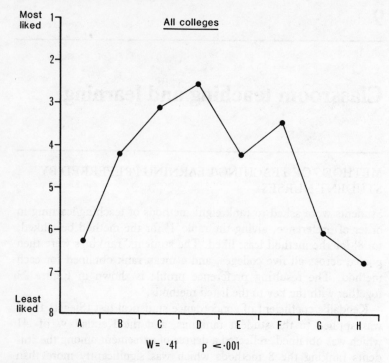

Fig. 23 Pre-experiment: students. Preference profile — methods of teaching/learning

Key: A = Formal lecture
 B = Lecture with time for questions or discussion
 C = Small group tutorial (college)
 D = Ward tutorial
 E = Practical class which includes demonstration
 F = Practical class which includes demonstration/practice
 G = Guided study
 H = Self-directed study

marked central tendency, with the mode residing, albeit narrowly, in the 'fairly often' category. In Colleges IV and V the mode was clearly in the 'rarely' category, with 23 (77%) of College IV respondents and 13 (62%) of College V respondents giving this response.

All teachers are aware that students — be they nurses or otherwise — and different classes within the same student groups, tend to vary in regard to participation. Undoubtedly some methods of teaching, such as the small group tutorial, encourage class participation more than do others, e.g. the formal lecture. It was not within the scope of this research to examine the teaching methods used in the colleges prior to the experiment. However, an example of the methods used with both control and experimental groups of students in one college of the main study is given on page 114.

Relationship of college teaching to ward practice

Two questions looked at the teaching given in college — was it helpful when students were working on the wards and did it relate well to nursing as it was practised on the wards?

In all, 113 students (95%) felt college teaching was helpful when they were working on the wards. It would have seemed reasonable to assume that, if college teaching was helpful, it would also relate in a positive way to nursing practice. However, this was not so for 75 students (63%) who considered it did not relate well to practice.

10

Theory and practice

EXAMPLES OF PRACTICE WHICH DIFFERED FROM TEACHING

Students were asked whether they could recall instances where their own ward nursing practice had differed from the taught method. From all five colleges, a total of 71 students answered in the affirmative. The numerous examples which they cited were categorised, as in the Nuffield Job Analysis (1953), into basic, technical and affective nursing:

> *basic nursing*... those nursing duties having their origin in the physical needs of the patient. (p. 27)

> *technical nursing*... all nursing tasks that are concerned with the treatment of the disease from which the patient is suffering. (p. 37)

> *affective nursing*... social and psychological needs which have their origin in the fact that the individual has to adjust himself to his changed circumstances. (p. 28)

Table 8 gives the number of comments in these three categories.

In the category of basic nursing, daily hygiene needs, especially bed-bathing received by far most comment:

Table 8 Pre-experiment: students.
Recalled examples of practice which differed from what was taught

Nursing work performed differently from way taught	Colleges					Total of comments	
	I	II	III	IV	V	N	%
Basic nursing	13	3	4	9	3	32	42
Technical nursing	12	5	9	7	8	41	53
Affective nursing	2	-	1	1	-	4	5
No. of comments	27	8	14	17	11	77	100%

In college you are taught to wash the patient in a particular order and change the water half-way through. This is rarely done on the ward.

Failing to give bed-rest patients a basin at night for hands and face, or basin for hands after using commode.

There was evidence in several comments that the respondents, a majority of whom were junior students, had failed to grasp principles (or may not have been taught principles) and their adaptation to different patients' individual needs, e.g. again re bed-bathing:

The patient was given a basin of water and told to wash areas he could reach himself and the nurse would wash his back and other areas he could not reach.

Oral hygiene — using gloves instead of dressed artery forceps.

However, there was also evidence of the persistence of soap and water methods of giving pressure area care, in spite of a number of research findings to contra-indicate this.

Pressure care — in wards the only way is patients get bottom rubbed with soap and water, when we were taught to do two—hourly turning of patients.

In the category of technical nursing, 41 examples were given and they included evidence of both careless, and at times dangerous practice in the wards:

Nasogastric feed — taught to introduce slowly — a *senior* member of staff showed the procedure and supervised me. The feed was introduced in a 50 ml syringe and she used the plunger to *push* the feed in (student's *underlining*). I only used that method once.

Recently three senior members of staff showed dressing technique, all three different and one definitely not aseptic.

Doing the medicine round, the nurse handing out drugs rarely, if ever, waits to see the patient swallowing the tablets.

In a number of comments, such as the latter, reference was made to details of care such as a student could very easily do, or not do, as she herself decided. There was obvious influence from what was seen to be done by others, i.e. the students might be said, in several cases, to be simply conforming, rather than acting in a thoughtful way.

Temperature taking, dressings and the giving out of medicines received most comment in the technical nursing category, but also mentioned were procedures such as catheterisation, and catheter hygiene, intravenous infusion, taking of blood pressure, care of chest drains, application of Kaolin poultices and many others. It was noted that, in regard to both basic and technical nursing, all respondents mentioned only procedures. There was no evidence of care of the individual patient *per se*.

There was little comment on nursing which could be categorised as referring directly to social and/or psychological needs of patients (an interesting comment in itself, on both the teaching and the practice of nursing). Two of the four comments received were:

> In college always taught to give patient complete privacy — on wards half the time it is not possible.
>
> Carrying out a procedure regardless of protests and with no explanation.

Seven students mentioned 'lack of time' in the wards:

> There tends not to be enough time on the wards to do everything by the book.
>
> Bed-bathing — the way we are taught takes too long when there are half a dozen more patients still to do, and we are often reprimanded for taking too long bed-bathing or removing stitches.

Such comments may reflect differing priorities betwixt ward sister and teacher or possibly somewhat idealistic teaching, e.g. 'There is not so much rigmarole in the method used on the wards as there is in college.

STUDENTS' OPINIONS ABOUT INTEGRATION

Some students viewed integration of theory and practice as a *college responsibility* mainly in terms of timetabling or ordering of theory before practice:

> Learning the aim of theory behind the practice and then using the skill with the patient soon afterwards.

For others, integration was a *student responsibility*:

> Doing practical nursing work while remembering the theoretical part, i.e. why it's being done and the correct way of doing it.

In this category, several students mentioned that integration aimed to achieve better patient care, e.g. 'translating or putting into practice what we've learned in college to benefit the patients.'

Where basic and technical nursing were practised as they were taught, theory and practice were said to be well integrated by students from all colleges, and also where specific links existed between the two environments of college and hospital e.g. — where students, *while* students, were taken from one place to the other:

> In Block I, we were given notes on bed-bathing and then were taken to a ward for a morning to bed-bath a patient.

Here theory was taught and followed by practice — a timetabling exercise or teaching method perhaps, but college-instigated. Integration was said to be good when college teaching promoted understanding when working on wards, and when ward tutorials were given which linked to what had been taught in college.

Understanding was important for many respondents, albeit mainly of reasons for procedures, than of how an individual patient might feel or of how or what they might explain to him:

> Biology and care of a person who has had an operation and a colostomy — no good if you don't know how and why it was performed.

However, for one student, well integrated theory and practice was linked to understanding of individual needs:

> Theory opens your eyes to needs of the patient which I might not have noticed, e.g. need for explanations . . . helps me think of what the patient will feel like with the different disorders.

From College III, 15 of the 31 senior students, the only students in the sample to have experienced the Block system *and* Study Days all within a modular programme, commented very favourably on their experience of obstetrics and community care, when Study Days were the method of organising the theoretical component:

> We were applying what we were taught immediately afterwards, by spending one day per week in college and then practising on the wards and in the community.

Students' perceptions of a lack of integration between theory and practice were expressed in many examples which were the obverse of those given above, e.g. where practice was not depicted realistically in the teaching:

> Care of pressure areas, the passing of nasogastric tubes when practice on a dummy is impossible.

I think the administration of intramuscular injections was a complete shock to us, from doing it with a piece of sponge and then going on to the wards and doing it to a real patient.

The difficulty of portraying reality from the college was well expressed by the following respondent:

Everything is easy to talk about in a warm friendly classroom, but having to do certain procedures can prove embarrassing or difficult, e.g. assisting with last offiices — very hard to come to terms with.

Where there was a lack of any physical link between college teaching and ward practice, where practice did not follow relevant theory:

It is not well integrated when we are given theory in school and cannot follow it up by going to the ward to practise.
I was giving injections, passing nasogastric tubes, checking insulin and many more such nursing practices, then I went into Block and got the theory of all these things. (A student who had a 4 week Introductory Block.)

Other examples of lack of integration were when ward staff appeared to the student to be unaware of her stage of training and experience, i.e. of what she might or might not be able to do; when tutors appeared to be 'out of touch'; and when there seemed to be conflicting values betwixt the school and the ward:

Every patient should be given individual attention and if there are problems he/she should be able to talk to the nurse — however, the nurse has no time to talk to the patient on this level at all.
I must always be doing something — instead of spending more time getting to know the patient.

Students were asked to suggest ways in which integration might be improved, and although no respondent was aware of the research experiment at this point, nor had any knowledge of the objectives which had been formulated, there was a remarkable similarity between students' suggestions for improvements and these objectives.

Students' suggestions fell into four main areas: (1) measures to link theory and practice in organisational (timetabling) terms, and in teaching methods; (2) measures to improve supervision, teaching and communication while the student was undergoing her practical experience; (3) increased liaison generally between college and ward staff; and (4) movement of people between the two places, i.e. college and ward in order to reduce the gap between what was taught and what was practised.

The greatest number of comments, 45 in all, were concerned with linking theory and practice:

> During block, nurses should be taken to the wards to see patients, suffering from diseases. They could be taken in small groups and the others could study in the college until they are taken. This could be done over a few days.

There were 24 comments about supervision and teaching during the practical component of training:

> More time should be given to the student while working on the ward, more clinical visits and help while working on the ward.

Liaison between college and ward brought 20 separate comments:

> By allowing all nursing staff, trained staff, sisters and nursing officers, to have seminars with the college staff on certain aspects of nurse training from time to time, along with the nurses in training, e.g. day courses.
>
> Nurse tutors should go out to work on the wards for short spells to see exactly how things are being done.

Other ward-related measures were felt necessary, such as meetings between senior and junior staff to discuss patients' conditions and progress, and maintenance of higher standards by ward staff, although three students felt maintenance of standards was a personal responsibility.

11

Ward teaching and learning

Ward teaching and learning was paramount for most students. They felt, by a 77% majority, that when college and ward were compared, the ward was the place where they learned most. They also ranked as their 'best-liked method' of teaching and learning, the ward tutorial.

It was also established, with virtually unanimous agreement (only one dissenting voice) that the student nurse should receive teaching while working on the wards, i.e. in the apprenticeship part of her training. It may seem strange to some readers that this question was even asked, but it was felt that there might be some, in the profession, who did not agree that this should be done. This was thought to be a possibility because of the recurring appearance, in the nursing journals, of complaints by learners about the dearth of ward teaching, and that little encouragement was given to students to ask questions on some wards. However, there was no evidence at all of doubt about whether ward teaching ought to be given, in so far as this particular sample was concerned.

The question of student nurses going from college to the wards, i.e. as supernumerary students under college staff supervision, there to undertake nursing practice, also received approval from 89% of ward staff and 88% of teachers.

Ward staff commented on the advantages to the students' learning which they considered would accrue from such directly linked college and ward teaching, although some raised doubts that the presence of the supernumerary students and their teachers could upset ward routine, upset patients, or deny experience to students currently on the ward staff. The teachers, on the other hand, while endorsing this method of organising ward teaching, on educational grounds, raised doubts about its feasibility in terms of supervision by teachers, given the present teacher/student numbers.

STUDENTS' EXPERIENCE OF WARD TEACHING

Students were asked about their experience of ward teaching, while working in general medical or surgical wards, firstly with regard to having received supervision or practical demonstration, and secondly with regard to tutorials.

(a) Supervision and/or practical demonstration

Students had received supervision and practical demonstration from all five staff groups, listed in their questionnaire i.e. ward sister, staff nurse, nurse tutor, clinical teacher and other student nurses. The students adjudged the frequency of such teaching sessions, and their opinions were summarised in Table 9. It was apparent from that Table that the category of 'never' accorded to the nurse tutor was an emphatic feature of the results from all colleges. There was slight variation of between-college opinion in regard to the contribution of the other staff groups, but the only other trained teacher, the clinical teacher, was considered to be carrying out very little supervision in Colleges IV and V especially — 81% of College IV respondents and 95% of those in College V said the registered clinical teacher was rarely or never supervising. In both these colleges, the 'other students' were seen to be contributing a great deal to supervision and demonstration. In all colleges, the staff nurse contribution was consistently high.

The opportunity was given, in the questionnaire, to add 'other' grades of staff, and 27% of the sample (32 students) mentioned receiving supervision or demonstration from the enrolled nurse. Those respondents came from four of the five colleges, the only exception being College I. An attempt was made by the researcher to assess the proportion of enrolled nurses vis-à-vis registered nurses on the ward staff of the various hospitals by inspecting the trained staff numbers on the off-duty sheets available to her. However, this attempt was not successful, as the designation of staff nurse or enrolled nurse was not always stated. The researcher's subjective impression was that there were more enrolled nurses in the two hospitals attached to College III than in any other hospitals in the study.

Supervision by the doctor was noted by 19 students, the majority of whom came from College III. This was perhaps related to the fact that the College III students were part way through their third year of training. As the most senior students in the sample, they were likely to have the opportunity to work with the doctor more frequently than students in their first year of training.

Table 9 Pre-experiment: students.
Frequency of supervision/practical demonstration received

Grade of staff providing supervision	Frequency of supervision in colleges																				Response totals
	I				II				III				IV				V				
	A	B	C	D	A	B	C	D	A	B	C	D	A	B	C	D	A	B	C	D	
Ward sisters	1	6	12	8	4	2	1	1	0	9	19	2	2	13	4	14	2	8	6	5	119
Staff nurses	18	9	0	0	7	1	1	0	7	17	6	0	1	13	16	1	6	9	5	0	117
Nurse teachers	1	1	2	22	0	2	1	6	0	1	3	24	25	0	0	4	1	0	2	17	112
Clinical teachers	4	16	7	0	2	6	1	1	1	15	14	0	15	5	1	10	0	1	17	2	118
Other student nurses	9	11	6	1	4	2	3	1	6	9	12	3	0	7	22	1	11	8	2	0	118
Enrolled nurses	0	0	0	0	2	0	0	0	0	10	4	0	3	2	7	0	3	1	0	0	32
Doctors	0	1	3	0	1	1	0	0	0	5	7	0	0	1	0	0	0	0	0	0	19

N ≠ 119 in all cases, due to non-response to some parts of the question

Key: A = Often   C = Rarely
      B = Fairly often D = Never

Attachment of a weighted score to the frequencies
Although the frequencies of 'often', 'fairly often', 'rarely' and 'never' in this question were unlikely to represent equal intervals, a score or value was attached to these frequencies, as undernoted:

often	= a score of 3
fairly often	= a score of 2
rarely	= a score of 1
never	= no score

Thereafter it was possible to calculate a percentage score for each staff category in regard to their perceived contribution to supervision and practical demonstration. This calculation was done as follows — of 119 responses to the frequency of supervision by the ward sister (see Table 9) the actual score was 157. The 'best possible' score, had the ward sister received 119 ratings of 'often', was 357, thus the percentage score was 44%. Figure 24 below indicates the contribution of the listed staff categories using the weighted score. The registered nurse tutor, the staff member who had had most resources spent on the development of her skills as a teacher, remained at the bottom of the league, clearly not, in the view of the students, contributing to the teaching in the wards, where the students spend most of the 118 weeks of the practice component of their education and training programme. The clinical teacher, whose *raison d'être* is ward teaching, was making virtually the same contribution to that teaching as the ward sister.

(b) Ward tutorials
In an identical format, students were asked about the frequency of teaching or tutorial sessions received while they were working on the wards. The pattern of response was very similar to that for supervision. As shown in Table 10, in Colleges IV and V the clinical teacher contribution was again low — 94% of responses in College IV and 89% in College V were 'rarely' or 'never'. The clinical teacher contribution, however, was also low in College I, where 73% of responses stated 'rarely' or 'never', yet this was a college with a relatively high proportion of clinical teachers on the college staff (see Table 6). Also in College I, the staff nurse was noted to give tutorials considerably more often than the ward sister. There was a similar, though not so marked trend, in Colleges III and IV.

Attachment of a weighted score to the frequencies
When the same weighted score, or value, was given to the frequencies for tutorials, as was done to the above-reported findings on

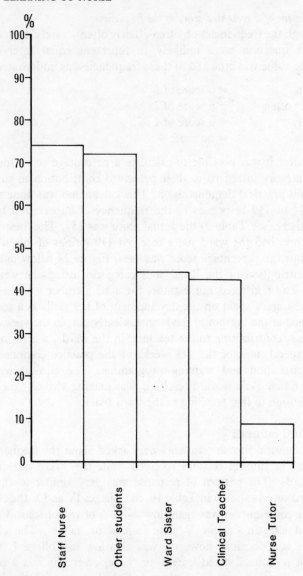

Fig. 24 Pre-experiment: students. Weighted score contribution to ward supervision/practical demonstration by listed staff grades

supervision and demonstration, an identical ordering of each grade's contribution was seen, although the 'other students' were shown to be using this method of ward teaching to a lesser extent than were the staff nurses (see Fig. 25).

Table 10 Pre-experiment:students.
Frequency of tutorials received

Grade of staff providing tutorials	Frequency of tutorials in colleges																			Response totals
	I				II				III				IV				V			
	A	B	C	D	A	B	C	D	A	B	C	D	A	B	C	D	A	B	C	D	
Ward sisters	4	1	13	9	1	4	4	1	2	6	15	7	8	10	10	2	0	6	5	9	117
Staff nurses	14	7	6	0	1	4	5	0	3	15	12	0	11	15	3	2	1	6	4	8	117
Nurse teachers	0	0	0	23	1	1	1	6	0	0	0	28	0	1	4	26	1	0	2	15	108
Clinical teachers	2	5	16	3	2	3	5	0	2	20	7	1	1	1	11	16	0	2	12	4	113
Other student nurses	3	6	9	8	0	4	4	2	2	3	10	15	12	10	6	3	2	7	7	4	117

$N \neq 119$ in all cases, due to non-response to some parts of the question
Key: A = Often C = Rarely
  B = Fairly often D = Never

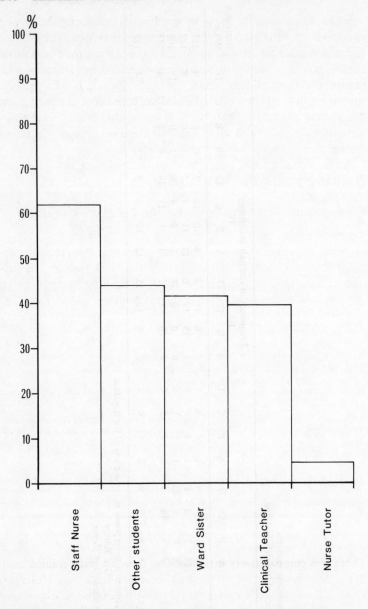

Fig. 25 Pre-experiment: students. Weighted score contribution to ward tutorials by listed staff grades

It should perhaps be borne in mind when examining the results in relation to ward teaching that there were many more staff nurses and student nurses in the wards than there were ward sisters or clinical teachers. It was the staff nurses and other students who carried out most of the nursing care of patients. It was perhaps surprising that no student mentioned supervision or teaching from the nursing auxiliary — another staff grade where relative numbers were high and where much of the working day was spent in direct patient care.

A few students (8%) commented on the variation in the amount of teaching given in the different wards.

Involvement of ward trained staff in ward teaching of students

Teaching in own wards

Of ward trained staff only 2 (both staff nurses in Hospital I), indicated no involvement in teaching within their own wards. The pattern of response, in terms of frequency of teaching, was similar in all hospitals and results were therefore amalgamated in Table 11, from which it can be seen that 92% of ward trained staff considered themselves to be teaching often or fairly often.

Table 11 Pre-experiment: ward trained staff.
Frequency of teaching in own ward

Frequency of teaching	Ward sister	Staff nurse	Enrolled nurse	Frequency totals
Often	40	67	5	112
Fairly often	24	60	8	92
Rarely	2	14	-	16
Never	-	2	-	2
Total respondents	66	143	13	222

Teaching in other wards

There was comparatively little teaching done by ward trained staff in wards other than their own. Only six respondents from Hospitals I and III considered they taught fairly often in other wards — one sister, three staff nurses and two enrolled nurses. Twenty five respondents from all hospitals and all three staff grades acknowledged teaching in other wards, but rarely. The only explanation offered as to the form of this 'other ward' teaching was that occasionally tutorials were given on 'chosen subjects' to students from a small number of adjacent wards or from a unit, e.g. 'cardiac arrest'.

Methods of ward teaching utilised by ward staff

Overall, the most popular method of ward teaching was supervision and practical demonstration. A close second choice was the tutorial and less frequently reported were teaching by example and teaching during the giving of the ward report. No one grade of staff was found to favour any one particular teaching method. There were 321 separate instances given — a very full response in explanation of ward teaching.

Teaching by supervision and/or practical demonstration was used by all three grades of staff and was mainly explained with reference to nursing procedures:

> Give practical demonstrations of surgical techniques. Supervise nursing procedures. (*SN*)
>
> By practical demonstration of procedures, e.g. dressing, pre- and post-operative care, passing of nasogastric tubes etc. (*SN*)

Tutorials, also used by all three grades, were sometimes on procedures or conditions, e.g.:

> Tutorials on basic subjects and items particular to the ward, e.g. peripheral vascular disease. (*SN*)

In addition a number of responses in this category referred to the patient rather than a procedure, e.g.:

> We discussed a certain patient who has undergone surgery. We start with the anatomy right through the pre- and post-operative care, until the patient is discharged. This way they can relate their lectures to practical nursing. (*WS*)

There was minimal evidence of organised planning of teaching sessions, and many mentioned the influence of time, especially with regard to tutorials:

> Give tutorials when ward is quiet — about conditions of patients in the ward at that time. (*WS*)
>
> Occasionally give tutorials about cardiac monitoring or cardiac arrest to staff from other units. (*WS* — one of the few who was also teaching in 'other wards'.)

Teaching by example was not often elaborated upon, however, teaching at report-time had a more articulate devotee:

> Giving a full report and teaching session when giving the ward reports. Giving time for discussion with all grades of staff at this time. I feel the Ward Report is a very important teaching factor. (*WS*)

This particular method was mainly mentioned by the ward sister grade. Only 2 staff nurses and one enrolled nurse said they taught by means of the Report.

Teaching by example was perhaps the method least likely to be appreciated, or seen as teaching, by some learners.

> I teach by example all the time. (*WS*)
> Teach general nursing care by example. Answer questions as asked. Explain procedures as they occur. (*SN*)

Such methods depend, for their use and their usefulness, upon the learner being able, or feeling free, to ask the question or to *see* the example. Also it is hardly realistic to expect that a 'good' example can be set at all times.

Involvement of tutors in ward teaching

Only three tutors considered that they taught often in the wards, 8 taught fairly often, 20 rarely, and 11 not at all. The proportion of tutors in the often and fairly often categories, compared to those in the rarely or never categories were 1 : 5 in Colleges I and III, and 1 : 3 in the other three colleges. (The clinical teacher was not asked how often she was teaching in the ward.)

There was no discernible pattern to the tutors' ward teaching commitment in any of the colleges. Five tutors worked always in the same ward or unit, but the rest worked in a number of wards, some made it their practice to follow students to whom they were personal tutor to wherever the student happened to be working. Others confined their teaching to students who were on their first ward experience, or were attending the wards from Introductory Block.

Ward staff perceptions of frequency of college staff involvement in ward teaching

Ward sisters and staff nurses were asked how often college staff were involved in teaching student nurses in their wards.

Their responses conformed to the pattern shown in the students' results. Ward staff considered the major contribution by the trained teachers was made, not surprisingly, by the clinical teacher, and that the contribution of the tutor was small. There were two differences within an otherwise similar trend. In Hospital III, the tutor contribution relative to that of the clinical teacher was exceptionally low, and in Hospital IV, ward staff recorded both grades of teacher as sharing the task of ward teaching to a greater extent than in any other hospital.

Responsibility for ward teaching

Questions as to who should be responsible for the ward teaching of student nurses were addressed to ward trained staff and teachers. Responses showed considerable division of opinion, which is summarised in Tables 12 and 13.

Table 12   Pre-experiment: ward trained staff.
Responsibility for ward teaching

Ward teaching	Joint education and service	Education staff only	Service staff only	Response N
Main responsibility	78 (35%)	78 (35%)	68 (30%)	224 (100%)
Responsibility if no RCT available	9 (6.5%)	5 (3.5%)	123 (90%)	137 (100%)

Table 13   Pre-experiment: teachers.
Responsibility for ward teaching

Ward teaching	Joint education and service	Education staff only	Service staff only	Response N
Main responsibility	19 (26%)	32 (45%)	21 (29%)	72 (100%)
Responsibility if no RCT available	7 (19%)	7 (19%)	23 (62%)	37 (100%)

Of ward trained staff, 70% thought the main responsibility should be either that of the teachers or shared between teaching and ward staff, but 30% thought that it should be a ward staff responsibility, as did 29% of the teachers. An attempt was made to seek out opinions about the tutor, in this regard, as opposed to the clinical teacher. Each respondent who had named the clinical teacher as the person, or one of the people mainly responsible for ward teaching, was asked who should assume this responsibility if no clinical teacher were available. Of 137 ward staff, 90% felt ward teaching then became their responsibility. Likewise, of the teachers themselves, of 37 respondents 62% thought ward teaching was not the responsibility of the educator, but of the untrained teachers, i.e. the ward trained staff.

Should the registered nurse teacher teach in the wards?

Opinions of ward staff and teachers as to whether the tutor *should* carry out ward teaching were obtained by asking respondents to choose from four statements (abstracted from the survey interview data) the one which came closest to their opinion. The statements ranged from one giving strong approval to the tutor as a teacher in the wards, to a completely negative attitude. The statements were as follows:

a. I feel very strongly that tutors should spend some of their time in the wards teaching student nurses
b. I think it is quite important that the tutor should do some teaching in the wards
c. I am not sure that the tutor should teach in the wards at all
d. The tutor's place is in the classroom, not the wards.

A marked majority of both groups gave a positive response to this question; thus they seemed to consider that the tutor did have some role to play in teaching of student nurses while they were at work on the wards.

Why the registered nurse teacher does not teach in the ward

From the survey data, a list was compiled of possible reasons why the tutor does not teach in the ward. Each reason had been proferred by a registered nurse teacher (tutor).

Teachers in the pre-experiment sample were asked to indicate their own opinion, by ranking these statements, assigning from 1, for the most likely reason, to 5 for the least likely. If they completely disagreed with any reason, they were asked not to assign a rank.

The five reasons listed were as follows:

The tutor does not teach in the ward because:

a. College commitments prevent her doing so
b. Ward staff resent her presence
c. The creation of the clinical teacher grade has made it easy for her to opt out
d. She has lost contact with the reality of nursing care
e. She lacks confidence in her ability to cope in the ward.

Less than half the tutor sample in the pre-experimental questionnaire were prepared to agree with reason (d), i.e. that they had lost contact with the reality of nursing care, and only 55% agreed that ward staff resentment of the tutor's presence was a relevant factor in the non-appearance of tutors in the wards as teachers. Overall, a higher proportion of clinical teachers were prepared to agree with each reason, than were the tutors themselves.

With regard to the rank ordering of the reasons, both tutors and clinical teachers ranked as the most likely reason for the tutor not teaching in the wards, that the creation of the clinical teacher grade had made it easy for her (the tutor) to opt out of such teaching. Both grades of teacher were also in agreement that the least likely reason was that of ward staff resentment of the tutor's presence, and both agreed in ranking in third place that the tutor lacked confidence in her ability to cope in the ward. The possibility that college commitments might prevent the tutor from carrying out ward teaching was ranked second by tutors and fourth by clinical teachers, and that she had lost contact with the reality of nursing care, fourth by tutors and second by clinical teachers. There was thus considerable consensus by the two grades of teacher prepared to assign a rank, i.e. agreeing with the possible reasons why the tutor did not teach in the ward.

The role or function of the tutor *vis-à-vis* the clinical teachers as ward teachers

Ward staff were asked: 'Do you think there is any difference between the tutor's function as a ward teacher and the clinical teacher's function as a ward teacher?' From their comments, it was apparent that a large majority of ward staff perceived a clear division of role or function — the tutor was concerned with theory, the clinical teacher with practice. This was a striking finding — in that it occurred in varying emphasis, in 90 of 101 responses, a number of which also added that the clinical teacher should link theory and practice.

> I feel the tutor's function should be solely theoretical whereas that of the clinical teacher is obviously of a more practical nature in the ward situation. (*SN*)
>
> Tutors should concentrate on theory. The marrying of theory to practice is the function of the clinical teacher. (*WS*)

Some respondents saw the ways or methods of teaching as different:

> As each ward differs from another — the tutor is giving a general teaching, whereas the clinical teacher can perform specific treatments in one particular ward, e.g. preparation of patient before and after aortic surgery. (*WS*)

This view of the clinical teacher as a clinical expert was stated plainly by a few:

> Clinical teacher should be a clinical expert in the working area. (*WS*)

Two opposing viewpoints:

> There is a difference at present, but ideally I think their function should be the same. (*SN*)

and

> If there were adequate numbers of clinical teachers to provide the link between theoretical classroom teaching and the practical aspect, there would be few occasions for the tutor to be in the wards at all. (*WS*)

There was evidence of a somewhat unrealistic view of the college or classroom, perhaps pointing to the necessity to bridge the gap and increase communication between service and education.

> The clinical teacher is at ward level — amongst the interruptions and the complications. This is at nurse-patient level — in the classroom there is a situation of peace and calm all the time which does not always happen on the ward. (*WS*)

Comments from the teachers themselves endorsed many of the views given by the ward staff but gave more emphasis to the following: (a) the course preparation of the two grades was different, and thus (b) the teaching methods tended to differ, (c) priorities were different — the clinical teacher having no or few commitments other than ward teaching whereas the tutor had college commitments as well as ward teaching, and (d) the clinical teacher was the clinical expert.

Some comments from the teachers were:

> The tutor, unless a trained clinical teacher, has not been taught to teach in the ward area.

> The CT should be predominantly involved in the teaching of psychomotor skills. Tutors' function is to impart general principles.

A number of tutors, and clinical teachers, suggested one grade of teacher would be preferable.

> At present there is, (a difference in function) — by virtue of CT's current practical skills they are better at demonstrating these than most tutors. One grade of teacher would be better.

> I do not agree with two grades of nurse teacher but at the moment the 'CT' appears to concentrate more on manual skills and the 'tutor' more on theoretical aspects.

> We complement each other's teaching, perhaps just emphasise different aspects.

The role or function of the ward sister/staff nurse *vis-à-vis* the clinical teacher as ward teachers

Ward trained staff were asked whether they thought their function as a ward teacher differed from that of the clinical teacher, and 70% considered it did.

Priorities were said to differ between the two groups of staff. The clinical teacher was considered to have more time to spend with the student and thus more opportunity to plan teaching.

> My *first* priority is the patients. The clinical teacher's first priority is the students. (*SN*)
>
> The clinical teacher's responsibility is primarily to nurses and teaching, whereas the ward sister's is towards patients and ward management. (*WS*)
>
> The difference lies in the fact that trained staff may not be able to spend time in teaching due to work pressures, and my tuition tends to be 'ad lib' — the clinical teacher can however plan and prepare her tuition according to her assessment of the students' needs. (*SN*)

Preparation differed — the clinical teacher was trained to teach, whereas they were not and she was also in touch with the college of nursing, by inference they were not.

> She is trained to teach juniors — we are not. (*SN*)
>
> Time! — and he knows how to teach and put over his knowledge to nurses. Also, his experience, on the whole will be greater than most of the ward staff. (*SN*)
>
> CT — helps the nurse to bring together the theoretical and practical teaching in the ward situation. Mine — help the nurses to appreciate the day to day care and management of the patients' needs and progress of their disease, or improvement. (*WS*)
>
> She is a link with the students' classroom and is already known to the student — a form of continuity with the classroom. (*WS*)

Clinical teachers were asked whether they thought their function as ward teachers differed from that of the ward trained staff. Of 29 respondents to the question, 23 (79%) considered that a difference did exist.

The differences they instanced were very similar to those which ward staff had given. The registered clinical teacher wrote of her training in teaching as 'a distinct advantage', and linked this with the fact that her priority was the student. She mentioned her different approach to teaching, her use of different methods and her ability to link theory and practice. It was interesting to note the clinical teachers' suggestion of the theoretician/practitioner division of function in ward teaching between themselves and the ward trained staff, which had been a very marked finding in the responses of the ward trained staff in relation to differences in function between the registered nurse teacher and the registered clinical teacher. Clinical teachers also felt that ward staff teaching tended to be more superficial than their own, and that ward staff were often unaware of a learner's specific needs.

> The clinical teacher has undergone a course of teaching methods and related subjects, e.g. psychology. The teacher has a greater understanding of the learners' requirement and the individuals' previous theoretical and practical attainments. Ward staff frequently have their teaching sessions interrupted which is not usually the case with the clinical teacher.
>
> Their training for registration did not prepare them to be teachers; that role is traditional, vague and haphazard.
>
> It is *part* of the ward sisters' responsibility to teach student and pupil nurses and sometimes the teaching may be incidental to the work. The clinical teachers' main responsibility is to teach student and pupil nurses and any work done is incidental to the teaching. Many ward sisters lack knowledge of *how* to teach, therefore they function differently 'as teachers'.

There was some comment that although the ward sister lacked training in how to teach, her knowledge of the patient was often as extensive as the clinical teacher's.

> I find the ward sisters in my experience (also looking back to myself in this position) have not the knowledge/confidence to teach — often ask for advice from myself. Ward sisters lack the necessary training to become a teacher although their practical knowledge of their speciality is excellent.
>
> The ward sister/staff nurse do more teaching by example and demonstration. My teaching more often is by following up these demonstrations with a tutorial and answering any queries the learner may have concerning medical conditions.

Evaluation of the experiment

This part of the book is almost entirely devoted to the evaluation of the experiment by those who were involved directly. Also included, albeit briefly, are the experience and opinions of the control group students and of their teachers. One chapter is devoted to reporting the results of the tests and essays. In order to 'lighten the load' in that chapter for the reader who is not enamoured of numbers and calculations, and yet not frustrate those with mathematical leanings, all of the Tables, Figures and most of the statistical detail have been sited in Appendix B. A short chapter depicts the student nurses' study patterns during the period of the experiment, and this is followed by a brief postscript, when the experimental group students 'look back on it all'.

The experiment, although essentially an educational experiment, the evaluation of a method of teaching/learning, involved co-operation between both service and education staff, and students, and so no description of the results could be considered complete if it contained only the opinions of the students and their teachers. The opinions of the ward staff were of equal importance. The experiment took place over a very brief period, i.e. from four to six mornings in the various hospitals, and, although experimental group students and their teachers were involved continuously throughout the length of the experiment in their particular college/hospital, most of the ward staff respondents would have been involved for only some of these mornings. To offset the brevity of the experience upon which their comments and evaluation were based, was the fact that every respondent had first-hand experience of managing her ward while the experimental group students were at work there. Each respondent had been responsible for giving, and receiving, the report of the patients cared for by these students, and had shared in the decision about the choice of patients with the researcher and teacher(s). It was considered most important that post-experiment responses should constitute a report of actual experience, and not hearsay evidence, therefore ward trained staff who had been on duty, but *not* in charge of the ward while the students and their teacher(s) were there, were not given a questionnaire.

12

Active experiential learning in nursing: the experiment evaluated in the opinions of the participants

THE DIRECT PARTICIPANTS.

The students

There were 43 students in the main study experimental group all of whom completed the post-experiment questionnaire. Where the post-experiment questions were identical in both main and pilot study questionnaires, the opinions of the 8 experimental group students from the pilot study college were added to this analysis, thus giving a total of 51 students, as shown in Table 14.

Table 14 Post-experiment: students.
Composition of experimental group

College/hospital	N in Group	% of total N
Pilot	8	16
I	12	23
II	4	8
III	11	21
IV	8	16
V	8	16
All colleges	51	100

The ward trained staff

Post-experiment evaluation was completed by 58 ward trained staff — 29 ward sisters, 24 staff nurses and 5 enrolled nurses, distributed throughout the hospitals as shown in Table 15. Where questions were identical in both the pilot and main study questionnaires, data from pilot study ward staff have been included. These numbers represent a 95% response rate.

The 58 ward staff represented eight general medical wards (10 staff), and 25 general surgical wards (48 staff).

158

Table 15   Post-experiment: ward trained staff.
Distribution of sample by staff grade and hospital

Staff grade	Pilot	I		II	III		IV	V	Total per grade	
		A	B		A	B				
Ward sister	3	7	-	1	2	2	8	6	29	(50%)
Staff nurse	4	11	2	3	-	1	2	1	24	(41%)
Enrolled nurse	1	-	-	-	3	-	-	1	5	(9%)
Total per hospital	8	18	2	4	5	3	10	8	58	(100%)
% of sample from each hospital	14	34		7	14		17	14		100

Note: From this point onwards, results from the A and B hospitals will be amalgamated, as the numbers are small. They will thus appear as Hospitals I and III.

The experimental group teachers

Eleven teachers were involved in the experimental group teaching, eight tutors and three clinical teachers. The same questionnaire was issued to both grades of teacher. Two tutors and one clinical teacher were from College I, one tutor from College II, one tutor and two clinical teachers from College III, two tutors from College IV and two tutors from College V. There were two senior tutors in the group, one from each of the latter two colleges. Opinions of the tutor and clinical teacher in the pilot college have not been included as the data from the former was incomplete.

Both grades of teacher are reported as one group. It was an essential feature of the experimental teaching method that there was no difference in the role or function of the registered nurse teacher and the registered clinical teacher.

FITTING INTO WARD ROUTINE AND TEACHER ROLE

The experimental method of teaching and learning about nursing is described in detail on page 86, and was based upon the principles of active, experiential learning (Rogers, 1969); principles considered by the researcher to be particularly apposite in nurse education and training. As it transpired, it was also seen as such by the large majority of respondents in all three groups.

Effect on ward routine and ward staff

Crucial to the success of any type of ward teaching programme is that it should fit in with the ward routine. Recently, the term ward routine has been commented upon somewhat disparagingly and while, at times, it can seem to take undue precedence, it cannot be entirely dispensed with in the efficient management of a general medical and/or surgical ward. A fear expressed by both students and teachers — and no doubt in the minds of some ward staff — when the researcher first broached the possibility of carrying out the experiment was that it would disrupt ward routine. Therefore, ward trained staff were asked if they found the experiment in any way disruptive of ward routine. For 91% of the ward staff, it caused no disruption. Those 5 (9%) who found it did, instanced either (a) a delay in ward staff gaining the use of the bath/shower for their patients, or (b) an occasion when neither the students nor their tutor were considered to be *au fait* with the ward.

The students had been anxious not to cause disruption in the wards and several had mentioned this in preliminary discussions with the researcher. In the event, their fear that if the ward was busy they would be an upset to the routine was not borne out by the comments made. Rather, the opposite occurred in that the very few negative comments came from the lightest (in terms of workload) areas. As a result of strike action having reduced the number of patients in two of the hospitals, a very few students felt they were taking away experience from the ward student nurses and this may have been at the root of the following comment:

> Some ward staff were not over-enthusiastic, some were helpful but others seemed to resent our presence.

Most of the students felt they had been of help to the ward staff in that their presence on the ward led to some relief of the workload. A number added that ward staff seemed interested in and curious about the new method while others said they did not seem to notice anything untoward:

> For some reason or other I was quite surprised at the friendly atmosphere which was always there. Staff were most helpful.
> They liked the idea of the integrated nursing and teaching aspect.

One possible 'spin-off' effect was given by one student:

> I think they felt they had to be on their toes because the tutors were coming into the wards.

There were 25 comments from ward staff as to positive effects resulting from the experimental method. They too mentioned the slightly lessened workload, with consequently more time for other patients, and the added stimulus and interest from the presence of the tutor and the students in the wards, although one respondent said:

> Some were uneasy about the presence of the teaching staff on the ward, but this could help keep them on their toes. On the whole, quite interested in what was happening.

One of the charge nurses took a different view:

> It ensured we did not forget we had a teaching commitment.

Teachers noted nothing other than positive effects upon the wards and ward staff.

No ward work other than what had been planned

The spectre of 'pairs of hands' arose many times when the researcher broached the possibility of the experiment with college teachers and students. It was said that ward staff would 'use' students in the sense that it would be they (the ward staff) who would decide on the patients to receive care. Several felt that ward staff would ask students to look after very 'heavy' patients, in a sense that they would not take kindly to students as 'students', nor to teachers who had a say in which patients were to receive care from the experimental group students. In the event, none of these fears were realised. No teacher reported that any of her students had been asked to do work in the ward other than that previously arranged and directly related to their lectures.

Roles of registered nurse teacher and registered clinical teacher in the experiment

The presence of the two grades of teacher in nurse education has been a matter of professional debate and concern for some considerable time. It was intended that there should be no difference in role or function for the nurse tutors and the clinical teachers who participated in the teaching of the experimental group students, and responses to the relevant question confirmed that this was indeed the case in the two colleges where the two grades were involved together. In Colleges I, II and IV only registered tutors were involved.

All of the teachers considered it was an appropriate part of their role to teach student nurses in the wards in this supernumerary capacity and as a part of their Block programme.

The three clinical teachers were questioned about the amount of their college commitment during the experiment. Two were quite satisfied but one felt that he should have had more time in college and in formal teaching. Should the experimental method become a part of their college programme, all three clinical teachers felt that they had a role to play — one confined this to 'teaching my specialty only'; another said:

> I would like my function to be what it was during the experiment — I had a feeling of *teaching the whole nurse*! (Respondent's *italics*)

The eight registered nurse tutors were asked if they considered their course prepared them to do ward teaching such as they had done during the experiment. Three teachers, all of whom had undergone their teacher preparation at university, and none of whom had been clinical teachers, said their course had prepared them adequately. Five teachers, four of whom were trained at a college of education and one at university, said their course had not prepared them for ward teaching. Four of these five were registered clinical teachers and each said that a clinical teachers' course was essential preparation for teaching such as was required of them during the experiment.

Effect upon job satisfaction of teachers
Job satisfaction was enhanced for nine of the eleven teachers during the experiment, due to patient contact, to increased communication with patients, ward staff and students, and to closer working relationships with teacher colleagues. One said:

> I feel I had the best of both worlds.

Another:

> Teaching as it should be, directed towards the patient.

For one teacher, job satisfaction was diminished as she felt:

> A little frustrated that some things were not covered due to the time factor.

STUDENT LEARNING AND SUPERVISION

How much was learned?
Student were asked whether, by combining college and ward work as they did in the experiment, they thought they had learned more, less or just the same as with the usual teaching methods. (The reader who doubts that the experimental method differed from the

norm is referred to both the summary (Ch. 17) of this book, and to the various comments of this chapter.)

A total of 42 students (84%) felt they had learned more, as a result of the experimental method, 7 (14%) that they had learned the same, and 1 (2%) that she had learned less.

One who felt she had learned about the same amount as usual, said, cannily:

> I cannot really commit myself until I see the results of the test.

The student who felt she had learned less was one of only two who had not particularly enjoyed the experimental method of teaching/learning. Reference to this student's choice of teaching/learning preferences in the pre-experimental questionnaire showed that she had a markedly different pattern of response from that of the sample overall — her first, second and third choices were of college-based lecture methods. Her fourth and fifth choices were the two study methods. Her seventh or second last choice was of ward tutorials. For this student, therefore, the experimental course had deprived her of lectures whilst her class colleagues received them. What is perhaps surprising, is that among 51 student nurses, she was the only exception, and that there were no others who said the experimental method gave rise to less learning. This student's final comment at the end of her questionnaire showed that she valued college, and also reinforced her dissatisfaction with anything which reduced time in college:

> Why not allow 'school' to be school, where we can learn and study.

She also suggested, as a means of raising standards of care in the wards:

> The answer would be for all third year nurses to go through Introductory Block again just before qualifying.

Supervision of students

Experimental group students were supervised during their periods on the ward by their college teachers. One teacher supervised four students, who might be working in pairs in the same ward, or on occasions, individually in two wards. The supervision received by each individual student therefore varied quite widely from day to day, and depended mainly upon the needs for nursing care of her particular patient, and the student's own ability to give that care, but also, to a certain extent, upon her location *vis-à-vis* the other students.

A majority of the teachers and of the ward staff considered supervision was 'just right'. One teacher of the senior students felt that initially with this method of teaching, her students had required very close supervision but that they quickly grasped the different approach which permitted less supervision.

Thirty-two students also considered the amount of supervision they received to be 'just right.'

Of the three students who felt more was required, two were from the senior group in College III. Of the 15 who would have preferred less, all but one came from the students who had been only 6 to 8 months in training and had practical ward experience of only 2 × 8 week periods. The reasons given as to why less was required, were that supervision was not necessary for basic care (5 students), that it made the nurse feel self-conscious (8 students), and in some cases was detrimental to student/patient relationships. Two students who said they felt self-conscious under supervision had previously said that they disliked the closer involvement of the tutor, which was a necessary part of the experimental method.

Some answers were most revealing of the dearth of ward teaching 'supervision' experienced by these very junior student nurses:

At first it was difficult to work with supervision *because I am not used to it*, but it makes you more aware of yourself and the patient and gets rid of previously learnt bad habits. (Researcher's *italics*)

Supervision to do a bed-bath or dressing seemed to be a waste of time since we have been doing these sorts of things by ourselves for the last 7 months. (i.e. 2 × 8 week periods on wards, the rest in Block)

Supervision tends to make me nervous and therefore I can't talk freely with the patient. I don't think supervision is necessary for basic nursing care.

There were 13 positive comments, stating supervision aided learning and helped the student gain confidence:

Under supervision I noticed that I learned more and had reasons for doing things, whereas most of the time I've been in the wards I just did things just for doing them.

I felt I wanted to be supervised — tutors were very willing to do so, e.g. the removing of sutures, and I appreciated the fact that they trusted me and let me do my basic nursing care relatively unsupervised.

EFFECTIVENESS GENERALLY OF THE EXPERIMENTAL METHOD

Students were asked about the effectiveness of the experimental method of teaching/learning compared to the college-based methods. The method did place students in direct experiential confrontation with what was to be learned — for most (46 students) this was very effective, for two students, it was not, and three students were non-committal:

> I was able to understand better than I think I would have in the classroom. I was able to put a face to the disease we covered, remembering in the patient's words what he had told me.
> Everything is much clearer when you can . . . speak to patients who have had the condition/operation.
> For me, not as effective — felt a lot of it was irrelevant, i.e. an hour to bed-bath a patient taught me nothing about his ca. stomach.

The above comment indicated that many students do have to be taught to *learn how to learn* from their daily work with patients. Indeed some respondents wrote of their difficulties in seeing what there was to learn at the beginning of the experiment, but that this resolved after a day or two.

Most equated effectiveness with active experiential learning, with easier recall, and the fact that they were more involved with their own learning:

> This method of learning is very effective for me personally, as I can learn things easier when I see it in practice rather than just being told about it. Also I learned how to deal with the patient in these situations.
> It has stuck with me, e.g. less learning from books.
> Much more effective. I found it a lot more interesting and even studied a bit more at night and read up a bit more of what we learned that day.

All 11 teachers considered this an effective way to teach, and all commented upon their answer. Effectiveness was equated with more opportunities for active learning, with reinforcement of learning, and with the emphasis on specific and individual needs of patients. Reservations were expressed as to a lack of time with the patients, and a lack of continuity of care, in that the student was not able to care for the patient throughout the course of his hospitalisation.

Advantages of the experimental method

Most frequently mentioned by the students, 37 in all, was the method of learning. Among the many descriptive terms they used were 'seeing', 'doing', 'talking over', 'associating', 'drawing together', 'finding out' — in other words, the active learning:

> I liked being able to take care of one patient without being too rushed, and I liked trying to join up what I had been taught in class with what I was seeing on the ward.
>
> You could see what you were discussing which made the theory easily understood and easy to remember.
>
> It drew together all the nursing care and the theory behind it for an individual patient.
>
> It brought out all the simple little things that made everything fit in.

Active experiential learning was often linked with the opportunity for patient contact. There seemed little doubt that many students were in their element in the wards, and contrasted this favourably with the classroom alternative. This patient contact was mentioned by 28 students:

> Working with patients, letting them explain their condition and how they feel, instead of being lectured to all the time.
>
> The work with patients, and learning from their personal experiences, and the case notes, was easier than reading from books and was easier to understand.

There were 15 comments relating to the teaching method, i.e. the students enjoyed the smaller groups, the use of less formal teaching methods and the contact with the individual tutors:

> The idea of small study groups is good, as it encourages people to learn more, also they have to read more as they cannot hide behind others.
>
> I liked being on the wards with the patients, and also the discussion-type lectures which the students took an active part in.

There were in all 76 comments from ward staff about advantages of the experimental method, the majority of which referred to the enhancement of students' learning, e.g. (a) the student was supernumerary so could concentrate on the patient without pressure and without interruptions, (b) the direct patient contact gave the opportunity to relate theory to practice immediately, (c) faults could be quickly picked up and rectified, (d) the total patient care gave the nurse opportunity to develop more insight, (e) there was realistic practice, yet in a controlled situation and (f) supervision and teaching was available from a tutor who was primarily concerned with the student and the patient she was nursing:

> What is taught in Block can by very different to the nurse in reality. So before actually working on a ward the nurse can see exactly what, or very closely the tutor has been talking about and she can also see what difficulties can or may arise.
> I feel nurses would be able to recall their theoretical teaching if it were followed quickly by short sessions with patients directly affected by the particular illnesses they are currently being taught about.
> I feel it brought the nurse and tutor closer together working in a 'real' situation.

Several respondents felt the experimental method was of advantage to the patients, a point which is dealt with later in this chapter, and a few said it helped the ward by relieving some of the workload:

> More time for ward staff to attend to other patients, so helping ward nurses. Giving student more of an insight into total needs and care of patient, allowing patient to help in training of nurses and allowing patient to 'give'.

Teachers too stressed the advantages to student learning. The method made available opportunities for the student to *learn how to learn* from her work with the patients — a vital feature in nursing education:

> The learner has the opportunity to learn how to apply the principles of nursing care, and to learn to adapt the same to the individual needs of the patient.

Some teachers valued the closer relationship with the nurses, and the fact that the method made possible greater observation of the students' practical work, thus enabling the teacher to help the student more:

> Feedback much more quickly from nurses in relation to coordinating theory and practice. A chance to see at first hand and hear directly the attitudes of the learner to new situations. Closer relationships with ward staff.

Disadvantages of the experimental method
All three groups were asked about the disadvantages, as they saw it.

Of the students, nine found no disadvantages, and 11 did not like to get up early! Experimental group students began their day one to one and a half hours earlier than on a normal Block day, and therefore than their colleagues in the control group. They did of course have a correspondingly early finish to their day, but there would seem no doubt that one advantage of the Block system in the students' eyes, is that it provides a later start to the day. This seemed a very natural comment.

Lack of time was mentioned by 17 students, and there seemed little doubt that this was a problem for some of the students on some of the days. Even when two nurses shared the care of one patient, there were occasions when the students felt rushed.

> We did not have enough time to do everything we would like to have done and having to care for a patient only for two hours did not give us enough time to get to know him.
>
> There wasn't much time to look at notes, but that is really no great complaint as the patient told us most of the history.

The students were not only carrying out total patient care, but also had to read and then copy notes from the Kardex, and the patient's case history folder. For junior students, the latter was not a particularly familiar document. On a very few occasions, they were not familiar with the ward, and then it could take them a little longer to find equipment. Some of the students were carrying out care, such as dressings, of which they had no previous practical experience, and this therefore took longer than had they been skilled. The students who were concerned over lack of time were distributed evenly throughout all but one of the colleges. In College III, where the students were more experienced and senior, only one felt there was insufficient time to carry out the care required by the patients.

A feeling of a lack of security was reported by four respondents (3 from College I) as they had 'fewer notes' than normally. Conversely, five students said that there was too much writing to do — and they cited the completion of the nursing care plans.

There was no doubt that the existence of a control group, imagined to be continuously writing down copious notes, heightened the feeling of lack of notes for some of the experimental group:

> I felt a bit insecure about lack of notes/theory compared to the control group at first.
>
> There was not enough time to carry out everything that was

supposed to be done and all the screeds of notes that we were missing over in the school of nursing.

I felt that we had to do too much writing and that this part of the experiment was very tiring, although I did learn by writing things down.

Three students commented upon feeling ill-at-ease because of the presence of the tutor, e.g.:

Being with the tutors. They made me feel ill-at-ease and this I think affected my relationship with the patient. I do understand that they must be present.

A majority of ward staff found no disadvantages — one senior ward sister remarked only that 'the newness and all the staff took us by surprise'. There were in all 18 comments about disadvantages, seven of which mentioned that there was too little time spent with the patient, and that neither students nor patients had continuity, i.e. the same students did not always return to nurse the same patient on a second day. From three comments, it was revealed that the respondents were not really aware of the students' learning needs. One staff nurse said: 'The nurses will gain little idea of the work of the ward as a whole.' This was not of course the purpose of the ward practice for these junior students. One sister commented that the teaching was unrealistic: 'students are not part of the ward team and are getting an unrealistic time allocation for each patient.' — a sentiment which showed a certain lack of appreciation of the fact that the student was learning as she was working, and of the fact that extra time is essential if teaching and learning is taking place.

Whereas quite a number of the ward staff and students had seen no disadvantages in the method, all 11 teachers were aware of one or more disadvantages. Almost all were related to time. Eight of the teachers mentioned this aspect — not enough days in which to get used to the method of teaching and of learning, not enough time in the wards, not enough time when back in the college:

Students were just settling down to it when it was over. (This comment from the college with the shortest time of four experimental mornings.)

Lack of time — much of this due to my own inability to adjust the content of what was being taught.

Two teachers commented that patients were not always available with just the right, clear-cut condition at precisely the right time.

EFFECT UPON PATIENTS

Effect on patients directly involved

Most students (35) commented that patients appeared to enjoy receiving the individual attention and having someone interested especially in them, but also, and a sign of sensitivity by the students, 18 said that there were patients who seemed to enjoy giving, i.e. they felt proud and pleased to help. It was most interesting, that, without putting it directly into words, students referred not only to the fact that they were meeting the patients' very basic physical needs for care and comfort (and for some who were very ill and weary it was simply that), but also that for some patients they were meeting needs of a higher order (cf. Maslow). It appeared that, by means of this experimental teaching/learning method, needs for self-esteem, so often not met in hospital, were being met. Patients were enabled to feel useful, and important:

> I think the patients enjoyed it as they usually feel helpless, and I think they enjoyed being a part of something and helping.
> They enjoyed the attention, and they too were able to learn about their condition.
> The patients enjoyed the feeling of being useful, and they liked the total patient care and having the chance to talk.
> They felt very important because they could teach us.

Two other effects upon patients were noted (1) in the students' opinion, the patient was given a higher standard of care and in the main this was felt to be due to the lack of rush and to the individualised attention, and (2) in some cases, the students felt anxious lest they might have overtired the patient. In illustration of the latter point, one student said:

> Because I only had two hours, I may have exhausted the patient, because I wanted to attend to all his needs in these two hours.

This aspect was commented on by 5 students, and in each case they were referring to their care of particularly ill patients who had required extensive dressings as well as total basic care.

The comments to this question provided evidence to suggest that, simply by altering the method of delivery of patient care from the fragmented task assignment model to the total patient care model, students were enabled to become aware of, possibly more sensitive to the patients' needs for rest. The possibility that their own well-intentioned efforts to 'care' may have detrimental effects for the patient is less easy to observe in a task assignment method of organisation.

Ward staff and teachers commented in strikingly similar vein to the students in regard to the effects upon the patients.

Effect upon other patients in the ward

Because, in early discussions, the researcher had heard fears voiced about the effects of the experimental method upon other patients in the ward, principally that they might feel neglected, a question about this aspect was included in the ward trained staff and teacher questionnaires. These fears were not at all borne out by the reality: 46 respondents said there was no effect upon the other patients in the ward, that indeed many were unaware of anything untoward, six said the other patients benefited in that more time and care was available for them, and four that several patients seemed interested in and curious about what was going on. In each case, the latter comment came from staff in wards where there was a cubicalized design. The resultant closer contact between patients and staff in these areas, compared to the situation in Nightingale wards, meant that other patients, if fairly fit and alert, were more aware of what was going on and did indeed take an interest. On many occasions, especially towards the end of an experiment, the researcher found herself in conversation with all four patients in a cubicle, both hearing about themselves and being asked by them about 'the young lassies' as the students were often called.

One sister commented:

> No one complained of the patients having preferential treatment — most important.

TOTAL PATIENT CARE OR TASK ASSIGNMENT

Students in the experimental group at no time went on to the wards to carry out specific procedures or tasks *per se*. They went in order to give total nursing care, to patients whose disease conditions were such that they linked directly with the students' current lectures. Two criteria were equipoised in making the decision about choice and number of patients — the students' learning needs, and the patients' needs for care. After the experience of the experiment, students were asked 'if you had a choice between giving total patient care to a few patients, or giving patient care by task assignment, which would you prefer and why?'

There was an overwhelming preference for total patient care.

Only one student preferred task assignment. The remaining students (98%) who opted for total patient care, said this was better for the patients and also for the learners. They gave many comments 32 of which related to improved patient care, and 36 to enhanced learning for themselves. Again the value of experiential learning was emphasised. Students also said that total patient care increased their job satisfaction and facilitated the teaching of junior nurses. Students' attitudes to their patients were revealed in these replies. Many set a value upon individualised care, i.e. attention to individual needs, upon a closer nurse/patient relationship, getting to know the patient, taking time with patients, and in some responses, contrasted the two forms of delivery of care to the detriment of task assignment. Two students used the factory and assembly line analogy in relation to task assignment. All quotations began:

> I prefer total patient care because . . .
> . . . you get to know at least some of the patients this way; by task assignment — none of them well. Also task assignment tends to be less interesting.
> . . . you become more concerned and involved with the patient rather than the tasks to be done.

One student, while seeing the advantage to the patient in total patient care, also showed her awareness of the inherent risk for the student of becoming 'too involved':

> I prefer total patient care because . . .
> . . . we could learn the patient's needs and this would help the patient. However this would involve the risk of getting too involved with one patient.
> . . . you are more aware of the patient and you can meet his needs more fully as you see one need following on from the other. Also it is easier to meet his mental and social needs as you are communicating for a longer time.
> . . . as you could treat them more as individuals and get to know them better and you could carry out your own standard of nursing care to these patients.

These results indicated that, for some of the students in the experimental group, the affective objectives listed at the close of the learning objectives for the experimental course (see Appendix A) were achieved, i.e. they assigned a value to individualised care:

> I prefer total patient care because having done task assignment, it is very apparent that patients are treated more as an

individual with total patient care (not one number on a bathing list). They benefit more, in that the nurse has time to make more observations and the nurse then gets to know more about specific care of condition more easily.

ACHIEVEMENT OF OBJECTIVES

Student opinions
As a part of the evaluation of the experimental teaching/learning method, specific student-oriented objectives were presented to the experimental group students. They were asked to state whether the experimental method met these objectives 'more', 'less' or 'no differently' than other teaching methods which they had experienced in their nursing education. At no time prior to this had the students known about or seen these objectives. Their evaluation is given in Table 16.

Table 16 Post-experiment: students.
Achievement of objectives of experimental method

Objectives	More N	Less N	No differently N	Total N
1. Help *you* to relate theory and practice in nursing	48	-	2*	50
2. Prepare you to return to work in the wards	32	4	15	51
3. Stimulate interest in your studies	33	1	16	50
4. Enable you to take part in class discussions	38	-	13	51

* = All from College I

In regard to every objective, a majority considered they had been achieved. However, in relation to three of these objectives, the experimental method was shown to have been no different from other teaching methods for a number of students.

An important aim in all of nursing education is to prepare the student to return to work in the wards. Fifteen of the students felt the experimental method prepared them no differently in this regard and 4 respondents (all from College I) felt it was less effective in preparation. There was no evidence in the data as to why this method was considered less effective preparation for return to the ward by these students, although it did seem that for two, the paucity of their notes was a problem.

The fact that 16 students found it no more, and no less stimulating of interest than other methods may be because a majority of student nurses are, in any case, already interested in their studies.

For 38 students, the experimental method enabled them to take more part in class discussions. For 13 this was no different. Of the 38 who said they took more part, 30 had responded to the question about participation in class discussions in the pre-experiment questionnaire — three already participated often and 9 fairly often, but 18 had previously participated rarely. Of those 13 who evaluated this objective as 'no differently' seven were in any case often or fairly often taking part in class discussions, but six were rarely able to do so. For those latter students, therefore, the experimental method did not lead to any increase in their participation, in spite of the fact that more overt opportunity for participation was provided, (a) in the more informal methods of teaching which dealt with subject matter directly relevant to work the students had just been involved in, and (b) in the smaller group teaching.

The main aim of the study was that expressed in the first objective and this received a unanimously positive response in four of the main study colleges and in the pilot college.

Ward staff and teacher opinion

Ward staff and teachers were presented with the objectives of the experimental method of teaching/learning. Prior to receiving this questionnaire, there had at no time been any mention of these objectives.

They were asked to evaluate by expressing their opinion as to the degree of achievement or non-achievement of each objective on a six point, equal-appearing interval scale, (Tuckman, 1978) as shown below. A tick was to be placed in the appropriate box (Diagram A)

Positive			Negative		
+++	++	+	—	—	—

Diagram A

Their evaluation is shown in Table 17. The figures from the teachers are given in italics immediately beneath those from the ward trained staff. The last three objectives were evaluated only by the teachers.

Table 17   Post-experiment: ward trained staff and teachers.
Achievement of objectives of experimental method

Objectives	Positive				Negative		N
	+++	++	+	-	–	—	
1. Help the student integrate theory and practice	35 *5*	16 *5*	6 –	– –	– –	– –	57 *10*
2. Increase communication between tutorial staff and ward staff	16 *8*	18 *2*	20 *1*	1 –	– –	1 –	56 *11*
3. Lessen the gap between the ideal and reality in nurse education	23 *5*	19 *3*	11 *1*	1 *1*	– –	1 –	55 *10*
4. Bridge the gap between education and service	19 *6*	15 *2*	18 *3*	3 –	– –	1 –	56 *11*
5. Better prepare the student nurse for her ward work and responsibilities	21 *5*	16 *4*	14 –	3 *1*	– –	1 –	55 *10*
6. Improve ward staff's understanding of what a student nurse can do at various stages of training	8 *3*	19 *2*	17 *3*	7 *2*	– –	3 –	54 *10*
7. Improve standards of nursing by supervising the student nurse in giving planned and individualised patient care	22 *8*	19 *1*	11 *2*	1 –	– –	2 –	55 *11*
8. Diminish stress for the ward teacher by making the student nurse supernumerary	7	2	2	–	–	–	11
9. Diminish stress for the teacher by giving a measure of control in the choice of patients and consequently a measure of predictability of teaching	8	1	2	–	–	–	11
10. Diminish stress for the student nurse by making her supernumerary while she was giving care and being taught on the ward	8	2	–	–	–	–	10

N. B. Figures in italics indicate teachers' ranking.

Further analysis of the evaluation of the objectives was undertaken by 'scoring' the positive/negative scale as indicated in Diagram B, in order to provide a 'best possible score' of 6 for each objective from each individual respondent.

Positive			Negative		
+++	++	+	−	—	——
6	5	4	3	2	1

Diagram B

Thereafter it was possible to add the 'actual scores' from all respondents evaluating each objective, and to calculate mean scores to represent the evaluation by (a) all respondents from all colleges/hospitals, (b) respondents in each individual college/hospital, and (c) each grade of staff, i.e. ward sisters, staff nurses, enrolled nurses and teachers.

Firstly, with regard to the evaluation by the ward staff — this was a most encouragingly positive evaluation of the objectives of this method of teaching/learning, and was particularly important because, in the view of the researcher, no ward teaching programme can succeed unless it has the endorsement of the service staff.

The main objective of the experiment was to 'help the student nurse integrate theory and practice'. It was therefore most satisfactory that this objective was accorded the highest mean score, and that this score was compiled from a 100% positive response.

In the current situation in nurse education, where there is concern about 'reality shock' for the student returning to the wards from Block, it was important that the experimental method should be seen as a realistic rather than an idealistic preparation for nursing. It was therefore again very satisfactory to find that the relevant objectives were very positively evaluated.

It was also interesting to note that mean scores were tied in the evaluation of two very similar objectives — to 'bridge the gap between education and service' and to 'increase communication between tutorial staff and ward staff'.

The lowest mean score was given to the objective 'improve ward staff's understanding of what a student nurse can do at various stages of training'. Forty four respondents gave a positive evaluation, and 10 a negative. On reflection, the rather lower evaluation for this objective seems a realistic result, as ward staff involvement with the experimental group students was intended to be minimal and responses to previous questions in their questionnaire confirm that this was indeed the case.

Were the experimental method to come into use, it might be

that, as more students and teachers came to the wards — the students at differing stages and therefore caring for patients with differing degrees of dependency — ward staff would gain an understanding of what could be expected of students at the various stages of their training.

There was very little evidence of response rigidity in the scoring by the 58 respondents. Only four respondents made consistent use of a single column — one sister and one staff nurse scored each objective with one plus, and one sister and one enrolled nurse scored all with three plus. All other respondents used more than one column, and the negative scores were not consistently from any one individual.

Of the three staff grades evaluating the experimental method, the staff nurses allocated the lowest mean scores. Ward sisters recorded a higher mean score than the staff nurses on every objective. The enrolled nurses gave the highest scores. Secondly, with regard to the teacher evaluations — reference to Table 17 will show that teachers seldom gave a negative rating, and when they did, chose the single-negative box.

With regard to the first seven of the listed objectives, i.e. those also evaluated by the ward trained staff, the main objective of the experimental method 'to help the student nurse integrate theory and practice' achieved a 100% positive rating and a mean score only 0.1 lower than the objective 'to increase communication between teaching staff and ward nursing staff'. The latter gained the highest mean score in the teachers' evaluation of these seven objectives. Improvement of standards of nursing achieved the same mean score as the integration objective, which was a very satisfactory outcome, and next in order of scores came the objective dealing with the preparation of the student nurse for ward work and responsibilities.

There was only one exception to an otherwise uniformly high scoring of the objectives by the experimental group teachers. They, like their service colleagues, gave the lowest mean score to the objective of improving ward staff understanding of what the student nurse is able to do at the various stages of training.

Overall, their mean scores were slightly higher than those given by the ward staff. The group whose scores approximated most closely to those given by the teachers, were the ward sisters.

Objectives 8, 9 and 10, which were presented only to the teachers, dealt with the very real problem of stress associated with ward teaching, both for the teacher and for the student nurse. The teachers' evaluation showed that the experimental method was seen as a very effective way of diminishing this stress.

SUGGESTIONS FOR IMPROVEMENT

Teachers were more forthcoming than ward staff had been in regard to ways in which the experimental method could be improved, especially in regard to student learning and patient needs. The dominant note was of the need for more time — students it was felt would benefit from a longer period of time with the patients, as would the patients. Suggestions given were that students might remain in one ward for several days, returning to the same patient, or patients, on each day; that the time when they came to give care might be varied to take account of differing activities at different times of the day; that they might follow through care for patients with similar disease conditions but at various stages, e.g. on admission, pre-operatively, post-operatively and then when convalescing, if possible including the after-care of the patient.

Three of the teachers felt there was a need for more college time to be given to the seminars.

FEASIBILITY OF THE EXPERIMENTAL METHOD: CONTROL AND EXPERIMENTAL GROUP TEACHER OPINION

Teachers of both the control and the experimental groups were asked to comment on the feasibility or otherwise of the altered teaching method, as one possible method of teaching student nurses at certain stages of their training.

The researcher felt it was reasonable to expect that control group teachers would have formed an opinion about the method as, although they did not have first hand experience, they could not but be aware of what was happening, as they were in daily contact with the experimental group students and their teachers. All but one of the control group teachers considered it to be feasible, and approved the method. The difficulties they saw were in relation to the numbers of teachers they thought would be needed to put it into operation, and the problem of organisation when class numbers were large.

Opinions of the experimental group teachers in regard to feasibility were considered to be most important, based as they were on their direct experience of the method, albeit for a fairly short period. Apart from one clinical teacher, who felt she had insufficient knowledge about the Block programme to enable her to comment, all experimental group teachers considered the method to be feasible:

This method of teaching is possible at all stages of training and must be commenced in Introductory Block to set foundation for more senior learning experience.

One teacher intended to put the experimental method into immediate use, and another to discuss the possibility of its use, within a Management Block, with her colleagues in both education and service:

> It is feasible as a method of teaching student nurses while in Block, particularly post-registration nurses whose training is short. It would also be ideal for nurses in the pre-registration period to teach them what to look for as a staff nurse. I am going to use this method of teaching with in the first instance post-registration nurses doing general training.

The other respondent referred to above said that, although it would take a good deal of organisation with a large group, she believed it could be done, and added:

> I would be delighted to try this with ward management as well as patient care. This would require even more co-operation with senior ward staff.

Although three teachers mentioned the factors of time, staff numbers, and/or organisation, their approach was more pragmatic than that of their control group colleagues, no doubt because of the fact that they had experience of the method. One teacher said that with large groups the method could be used 'on rotation', i.e. some students in class and others in the ward for certain topics. Two felt that, as the GNC Syllabus stood at the moment, it would not be possible to cover every topic if teachers used this method of teaching to a great extent. This response of course begs the question — is it necessary, even advisable, to 'cover' every topic?

However, from the experimental group teachers, there was general affirmation of this method of teaching nursing; said one:

> We must not wait too long before introducing this method . . . when one considers how short the learner's clinical experience is, this method is invaluable in certain areas.

13

The experience of the control group students and their teachers

Those class members who had remained in the college of nursing, i.e. the control group, numbered 56. There was no control group in College III, and, as the questionnaire was developed only as a result of the experience of the pilot study, there are no data from the pilot college. Although there was essentially no change in their course content, or in the number of hours spent on the subject matter, it would have been unrealistic to consider the control group's experience to have been totally unaffected by the research experiment. The class size was reduced, and certain unusual features were imposed upon their timetable; in particular their nursing leatures were concentrated into a shorter space of time and took place during the four to six days of the experiment — for the control group this was, as a general rule, in the first two periods and the last period of each day — with slight variations in each college.

Given the opportunity, 37 (66%) of control group students would have preferred to be in the experimental group, their reasons, mainly, that they liked to learn by 'doing' or 'seeing'. Several students commented that they would like the opportunity to compare the two different ways of learning:

> It would be a chance to see if it helped me to learn more. It would also give me some idea how to approach patients with different conditions.
> I would like to compare the two methods of teaching and assess which I found most beneficial.

From those 17 students who preferred to remain in the control group, the reasons given were that they would have more notes, that they preferred what they were used to, and that they felt apprehensive if they did not know the outcome of something new:

> Compared with the experimental group, we have more notes to look back on in later years.

I learn better sitting at a desk with a tutor.

I'd rather be doing what I'm used to, the experimental group didn't know the outcome of this, and it is an important subject.

Two students, diametrically opposed in terms of the amount of work they themselves preferred, commented in regard to the amount of involvement and work they thought the experimental method required.

The pro-control group viewpoint:

I don't think I would like to take part in the experimental group as I feel I would have too much work to do on my own, therefore I would prefer not to take part.

The pro-experimental group viewpoint:

I feel that I would have enjoyed learning in a situation where I would be using the skills I have already and building on them in a real situation. I think I would be more involved in my education in the experimental group.

It is interesting that these two control group students, with only 'hearsay' knowledge of the experimental group experience, had comprehended and commented upon one of the fundamental learning differences between their own teaching/learning experience and that of the experimental group.

Students were fairly evenly divided in their opinion as to whether the research experiment had made a difference to their Block experience, apart from the respondents from College I where, by a majority of 11 to 3, students considered the experiment had made a difference.

Of the comments to this question, 21 gave evidence of positive Hawthorne effect, and 11 of a negative effect:

It made the Block more interesting — something different, which enabled you to concentrate more because you felt you were of importance and helping some people. It also made me study at night, which I probably would not have done if it was not for the experiment.

However, in College I, several control group students described their own experience as 'boring', 'too much information all crammed together', 'little attempt was made to vary the programme and teaching methods' and one student:

I think this experiment caused a bit of interference and upset to the class. Also I felt more resentment towards my work, I felt as though I was being cheated in my learning as I know I have great difficulty in learning anything from intensive formal lectures. I also felt that since it was an experiment then it wasn't so important to learn my work.

The type of teaching methods experienced by the control group students during the period of the experiment may have influenced their perceptions of whether the effects of the experiment were positive or negative. The only instruction which had been given to the control group teachers by the researcher was that they should carry on with their teaching of the subject using, as far as possible, the methods they normally used. In College I, 81% of the control group's hours were spent receiving lectures with some opportunity for question or discussion. By contrast, a majority of respondents in a college where a variety of teaching methods had been utilised, held a positive view of their experience.

Seven students commented upon the advantages of the smaller classes, and said this led to 'a better staff/student relationship', 'more personal'. One student expressed disappointment that, although the class size was reduced, no advantage was taken of this, i.e. no tutorials or discussions, and a laconic comment from one who felt the experiment made little difference:

> Block this time has just been the same as any other Block — except that the classes were smaller — and that was much better.

There were eight teachers involved with the students of the control group — five tutors, two clinical teachers and one uncertificated teacher. Four teachers found it an enjoyable and interesting experience, the others were less sure. One felt that it was no different from usual, and one considered it had been less enjoyable than teaching normally was.

Six teachers felt the experiment caused no disruption to the control group experience of this subject matter. Interestingly, and in line with the students' remarks quoted above, two tutors, both from College I, felt that there was disruption. One said the control group experienced boredom to some degree with the very long sessions, and the other that:

> they felt they were being 'saturated' with the one subject and at times seemed less receptive to the teaching given.

The effect of the experiment on the control group students was considered to be slightly detrimental by the two tutors in College I, because there was 'too much of one subject at one time'. Teachers in Colleges II and V felt the experiment had very little effect, apart from arousing some curiosity and the feeling amongst the control group students that they 'just might be missing out'; and in College IV a Hawthorne effect was reported, e.g. 'a competitive aspect which seemed to stimulate them and maintain their interest'.

14

Results of the tests and essays

(Relevant tables and figures are presented in Appendix B)

There were two parts to the evaluation of the test and essay scores obtained by the students who had experienced the experimental method — which combined supervised ward practice of relevant nursing with concurrent college lectures and tutorials — and the control method of entirely college-based teaching.

In the first part, the main and basic question was of the instructional effectiveness of the two methods of teaching nursing, and of their relative effectiveness *vis-à-vis* each other. The second part was concerned with the relationship between multiple choice tests and essays in nursing examinations, and with the reliability of the marking of such essay scripts.

The tests which are referred to throughout are the previously validated multiple choice (objective) test — which was identical at all three stages of the experiment, and across all colleges. The essays were identical at both stages at which they were used, but were college-specific. Although similar in content, as they were derived from the subject matter of the course as outlined in the General Nursing Council (Scotland) syllabus before referred to, the specific questions were not identical across colleges.

Scores on the test were calculated by a short programme added to the Rasch Item Analysis Model (Wright & Mead, 1977) which had been used for the item analysis when this test was constructed and validated. Scores on the essays were obtained by issue of all of the scripts to each of three neutral markers, all of whom were General Nursing Council (Scotland) examiners, i.e. they were responsible for correcting the essay-type Final State Examination scripts.

The detailed statistical analysis of the scores is presented in Appendix B on pages 240–252. The text of this chapter will therefore present only a summary of the test and essay results.

THE EFFECTIVENESS AND RELATIVE EFFECTIVENESS OF THE TWO METHODS OF TEACHING

The pre-test

The internal validity of the experiment rested upon the demonstration of effective pairing of the students in the two groups. Before any questions as to the effectiveness, or relative effectiveness of the two teaching methods could be answered, it was also essential to know, in relation to each student, her 'starting-off point', or baseline in terms of knowledge of the subject matter of the course. Pretesting was therefore a most important feature of the experimental design, as is discussed on pages 85 and 86.

The result of the pre-test showed a mean for the experimental group students of 52.53 and for the control group students of 52.63. There was no statistically significant difference between the experimental and control pairs (N = 32) on pre-test, and a high positive correlation between the two sets of scores was demonstrated.

The initial equivalence of the pairs of students in regard to knowledge of the subject matter of the course was therefore very satisfactorily confirmed by these results.

Demonstration of learning

The first and fundamental question to be answered, in regard to all the students, irrespective of group, was whether they had learned as a result of the teaching — whether their scores were higher at the end of the course than at the beginning. The answer was clearly positive. As measured by the difference between the post-test and pre-test results, for the by then 31 matched pairs of students, this first exposure to the course content resulted in gain scores of 15.86 for the experimental group students, and 14.98 for the control group students, a non-significant difference of 0.88 in favour of the experimental group.

Demonstration of retention of learning and/or forgetting over time

Retention of learning was demonstrated for students in both groups. For the, by now, 29 matched pairs of students, the gain score from pre-test to retention test in the experimental group was 16.47, and in the control group was 14.27. The experimental group mean was 69.00 and the control group mean 67.00, a difference of two points in favour of the experimental group. There was no evidence of forgetting over time for the experimental group, who demonstrated a minimal gain of 0.61 marks from post-test to retention test. There was very slight evidence of forgetting from the control group who showed a loss of 0.61 marks from post-test to retention test.

One further factor considered as of possible influence on test results at this stage of the experiment was the intervening practical experience of nursing for all students. This is reported later in this chapter.

At post- and retention stages, the essay scores were also available for comparison. The essays not only presented a totally different distribution picture from the tests, but yielded markedly lower mean scores. In the experimental group the post-test mean was 8.62 marks more than the post-essay, and in the control group it was 8.19. At the retention stage, the difference between the test and essay means was, for the experimental group students, 14.75 and for the control group students, 16.32. There were also clear loss scores betwixt post-experiment and retention of learning assessments — of 5.52 marks for the experimental group students and 8.74 for the control group students, a difference of 3.22 marks in favour of the experimental group.

Correlations of tests with essays

The obvious differences in mean scores between the tests and essays led to the question of whether the ordering of students was also different between the two measures, however, Pearson's product moment correlations were significantly high, indicating no great differences in the ordering of the students, within their groups, on the test and essay results.

In summary therefore, all students, whether taught by the experimental or the control method, had demonstrated by a gain in test scores that they had learned as a result of the teaching, and all had retained much of that learning over time. However, when essay scores were examined there was evidence of knowledge decrement over time. At both post- and retention stages, experimental group students were marginally, certainly not significantly better than the control group students. The next step in the evaluation was to look more closely at the differences between those taught by the experimental method and those taught by the control method.

Demonstration of differences

Firstly, the question was simply to establish whether, *within each pair*, the experimental student had achieved a higher score than her control partner on each of the post- and retention dependent variables. The Sign test for large samples (n > 25) was used (Siegel, 1956), but when positive and negative differences were counted there was no statistically significant result. Again, at post-experiment stage, the experimental group were fractionally ahead of the control group, although by retention stage the difference had widened considerably, though still it was not significant.

The final stage of the evaluation of the treatment effect made use of the more powerful parametric tests. The data, collected as they were in the form of scores, i.e. interval level, were suitable for such detailed analysis, and in particular, for the use of Student's t-test of the significance of the differences between the means. Where *within-pairs* differences were examined, as was done here, the efficiency of the randomised-blocks design came to the fore, in that it eliminated the inter-block or inter-pair variation, thus allowing the calculation of the standard error on the irreducible minimum within-block or within-pair variation. The larger value of t which resulted was very slightly offset by the reduction in the degrees of freedom which were calculated on the N of blocks (32) minus one, and not N (64) minus one. During the course of the experiment the original N of blocks of 32 was reduced, at retention essay, to 28.

The question now therefore was whether, at any point in the experiment, differences demonstrated by this small sample were of such magnitude as to be generalisable to the population of student nurses in Scotland from which the sample was drawn. The important limitation to generalisation of the results was that it was not possible to randomly select colleges of nursing, nor students within these colleges, to take part in the experiment. However, the allocation of students to experimental and control groups, following pairing of these students on their pre-test results, was a procedure which ensured random allocation to the two groups, controlled the variable of entering knowledge, and also ensured a spread of ability within the two groups of students.

The gain scores

Firstly, the gain scores achieved by students in both experimental and control groups from pre-test to post-test and from pre-test to retention test were tested for significance. The comparison was therefore between the same individual on the tests at the two stages of the experiment, i.e. she was paired with herself. As a gain, therefore direction was predicted, a one-tailed test of significance was used. It was concluded that student nurses experiencing either teaching method were likely to make a significant gain score between pre- and post-testing, and to retain a significant gain between pre- and retention testing, as all results were well beyond the critical value of t for the relevant degree of freedom. It appeared therefore that both courses of instruction were effective.

The loss scores

When knowledge decrement was examined by the same procedures as outlined above, the loss score on the tests was not statistically significant, for either experimental or control students, but was statistically significant on the essays.

The difference scores within each pair

At this point it was the between-test or between-essay difference scores for each member of each pair which were compared.

There was no statistically significant difference when scores were examined in this way, although again, it was interesting to note that, in the four comparisons which were possible, the experimental group mean difference compared favourably with that of their partners in the control group, and this was especially so with regard to retention of learning as demonstrated by the essay scores. Thus, the tren·¹ shown previously was maintained in this final and most precise test, although it was still not possible to demonstrate any statistically significant effect as a result of the experimental method.

Effect upon scores of relevant intervening experience of nursing

Finally, in this part of the evaluation, one important question remained. Was it possible to establish whether there had been any effect upon retention of learning as a result of the relevance or otherwise of the intervening practical experience of nursing on the wards? Relevance was defined as 'having nursed patients suffering from disease of the gastro intestinal tract during the intervening period betwist post-experiment and retention of learning assessment'.

Unfortunately, this comparison was not possible, due to the small number of pairs remaining (N = 3) when controlled on this variable. Abandoning the pairs comparison, and looking at the students in their groups, it transpired that 50% of the control group had had relevant experience and 50% had not whereas 68% of the experimental group had had relevant experience and 32% had not. The comparison which was made was of the between tests and between essays difference scores, within the groups, for those who had and those who had not had relevant experience. The t-test used was that for independent samples and the results showed there was no statistically significant difference between the mean differences for students in either control or experimental groups as a result of the intervening experience of nursing and its relevance or otherwise. There was, however, on each measurement, a tendency for those students who had had the opportunity to put their theoretical knowledge to practical use, to do better than those students who had not had that opportunity.

OF MARKS AND MARKERS

In this part of the evaluation, the teaching methods *per se* were no longer under scrutiny, nor was the treatment versus no treatment effect. Rather it was the relationship between tests and essays, and the reliability of the marking of essays which was examined.

Instructions to the three neutral markers from the researcher were to mark the scripts in the way they normally did when correcting Final State examinations. Two of the markers, Marker B and Marker C, were in the habit of constructing a marking key, which they then used to arrive at a score for each section of each script. Marker D was an impression marker, i.e. she read all the scripts through completely, then re-read each, section by section, and allocated an appropriate mark based on her impression of its 'worth'. She did not use a marking key.

None of the neutral markers would have been able to identify any of the students, nor was it possible for them to know which colleges were involved in the research. The initial 'A' was reserved for the markers in each individual college, who, in the interests of quick feedback of results to students, marked their own college scripts. However, as these markers were not 'neutral', i.e. knew which group the students were a part of, their marks were not utilised in the statistical analysis.

Essays, as tests, are frequently criticised, mainly on grounds of unreliability and subjectivity of the marking, as indeed of the setting of questions. The reason why the essay was used in the experiment was because it is in common use in nursing education, both as a measure of learning *en route*, and at the final examinations.

Relationship between tests and essays
The lower mean scores for the essays when compared to the tests, and commented on previously, were a constant feature whether the results were examined within colleges or across colleges. Correlations between these measures were however high, indicating a similar ordering of the students in the sample on both tests and essay results.

Inter-marker reliability or agreement

Because essay marking is known to be subjective, steps can be taken to try to mitigate this undesirable effect. Multiple judgments are recommended, and to a certain extent this was achieved in this research by the use of the three neutral markers, whose scores on the post- and retention essays were aggregated to produce an average score for subsequent calculations. This part of the evaluation looks at the characteristics of the marking by the individual neutral markers.

Marker D, the impression marker, gave the lowest mean score on both post- and retention essays. The most lenient marker on both essays was Marker B, who also made use of the widest range of marks. Because the marker means quite obviously differed, a one-way analysis of variance was performed, using the SPSS Program 'Reliability'. This showed that the difference between the means of the three markers was statistically significant.

The differences between the markers was further explored. There was no complete agreement between them on the score for any one student. The variation in the scores awarded to any one student was at times considerable, ranging from 33 marks to 1 mark in the post-essay, and from 34 marks to 1 mark in the retention essay.

As to the question of passing or failing, there was agreement between the three on 73% of the students for the post-essay, but on only 65% for the retention essay. The marker who had appeared most lenient on observation of the means, was displaced from that position by Marker C, who failed fewest students in both tests. Inspection of the scores showed this marker used the 50% mark altogether 19 times, over both essays, whereas Marker B used this score only 3 times and Marker D on 7 occasions. It was possible that where Markers B and D marked a doubtful student below the pass mark, Marker C gave her the benefit of the doubt, but that is only speculation.

In spite of all the differences between the actual scores awarded by the three markers, they were much more in agreement as to the ordering of the students. The Pearson product moment correlations between the markers, for the two essays, were very satisfactory.

It is relatively straightforward to re-adjust marks to correct discrepancies which arise from hard or easy marking — it would have been of much more concern had there been a low correlation between these three experienced markers of nursing examination scripts.

15

Student nurse study patterns

Throughout the course of the experiment, in all colleges, students kept a daily study diary. Since these diaries, from both control and experimental group students, were completed during the very abnormal circumstances of the research and the experiment, none of the findings presented below can be considered descriptive of student nurse study patterns in general. However, they did provide an interesting indication of study done, by this small sample of students, during a somewhat unusual time in their Block.

The sample who completed the diaries

Table 18 shows the sample of students whose completed diaries contributed the information for analysis, and the number of Block days and of weekends represented in the diaries. The sample included 43 experimental group students, 46 control group students, and 4 'others', i.e. class members who were undertaking RGN

Table 18 Number of students who completed diaries by college and number of days represented in the diaries

College	Students	No. of days of experiment	No. of Block days represented in diaries	No. of weekends in expt.	No. of weekends represented in diaries
I	27	6	159*	1	27
II	10	5	50	1	10
III	11	4	44	-	-
IV	24	5	119*	1	18*
V	21	5	103*	1	17
Totals	93	25	475*	4	72*

Note: The number of Block days (or of weekends) represented in the diaries was calculated by multiplying the number of students by the number of days of the experiment in each college (or by the number of weekends in each college). Discrepancies occur when a diary was missing for a day or a weekend from one or more students. This is indicated by an asterisk. An overall total of 6 daily diaries and 10 weekend diaries were missing. Response rate was therefore high — 547 diaries out of a possible 563 = 97%

training but were ineligible for the afore-mentioned groups because they had previous experience of the subject matter of the experimental course.

Officially designated study time
The proportion of available Block or classroom periods which were officially designated as study time was very small, as is shown in Table 19.

Table 19 Available classroom periods officially allocated to study

College	No. of Block days represented in diaries	No. of classroom periods daily	No. of total available periods	No. of total study periods	Study periods as percentage of total periods
I	159	6	954	98	10
II	50	6	300	34	11
III	44	6	264	8	3
IV	119	5	595	41	7
V	103	6	618	62	10
All	475	-	2731	243	9

The students in College III, where the proportion of study time was least (only 3% of the whole) were taking part in a one-week revision course, preparatory to working in their pre-registration period on the wards. All other students were in the course of an eight-week Block.

Of the 243 study periods, rather more were available to the control group students, than to the experimental group students. The former had 156 out of the 243 periods, and the latter 74.* In part this imbalance was due to the fact that very seldom was study time allocated to the experimental group students during the first three periods of each day, i.e. while the experiment was in progress, whereas there were several occasions when control group students recorded study time at that time of day.

Use of officially designated study periods
A majority of students in each college made use of the official study periods for study purposes, although only four students used all of these periods for the purpose for which they were intended, and ten used none. All four 'others' students were in the latter categ-

---

* The remaining 13 periods were available to the 'other' students

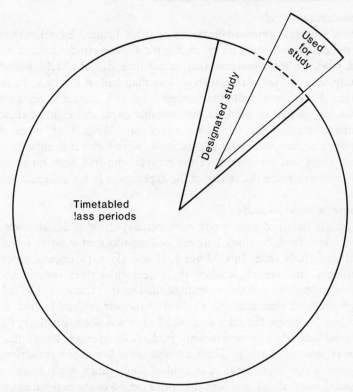

Fig. 26 Organised opportunities for study as a proportion of all class periods.
Excised section indicates use made of these study periods, over all colleges
Total class periods available = 2731

ory. Figure 26 indicates, over all colleges, the proportion of the total available class periods allocated for study, and the proportion of that time which was actually used for study.

The two colleges in which the lowest percentage use of study periods for study purposes was recorded, were College V and College II. In these two colleges, it was daily practice to designate the half hour immediately after the morning coffee break as a study period. This appeared to be a particularly unproductive period so far as studying was concerned. In many instances, it developed into an extended coffee break, which students were sufficiently honest to admit was not devoted to discussion which related to their studies.

When control and experimental groups of students were compared on this question, the former were found to have used 65% of their 156 available periods and the latter 72% of their 74 periods.

Self-initiated study

There were 244 reported instances of study being done other than at the designated study times, during the 475 days under discussion. Six students recorded that they at no time did any self-initiated study, and 34 that they did so on less than half of the experiment days. More than half the sample, i.e. 53 students reported studying on half or more of the available days, and eight of these students studied for some time every day. When both types of study, i.e. designated and self-initiated, were taken into consideration, there was no student in the sample who had done no study whatsoever during the course of the experiment in her college.

Time devoted to study

Students recorded total study time per day in minutes, and were not asked to distinguish between college-allocated time and self-initiated study time. In Colleges I, II and IV, experimental group students, on average, studied for longer than their control and other colleagues, and this in spite of the fact that there was less college-allocated time available to them to include in their figures. In College V, where the least amount of time was spent in study, the control and other group students studied, on average, longer than the experimental group. These average times however were arrived at from a very wide range of individual study times. Eight students studied one hour or less over the entire period of the experiment in their college, and five students studied for ten hours or more — the maximum period being 11.75 hours by a control group student.

Weekend study

The amount of weekend study done by students appeared, not unexpectedly, to bear a positive relationship to the occurrence, and proximity of an 'end of subject matter' assessment (an essay type of test). In College I, the weekend occurred after only two days of the six day experiment, the assessment was a full week ahead, and only 22% of students did any weekend studying — an average of 90 minutes each. In College V, where students completed the course on a Friday, the weekend and a public holiday intervened before their assessment, and 48% of students spent an average of 105 minutes each in weekend study. Students in Colleges II and IV, who had recorded the highest average weekday study times, were also those who studied most at the weekend. In both colleges, the assessment was scheduled for a Monday. All students in College II studied, for an average of 4.5 hours, and 75% of students in college IV did so for 2.5 hours on average.

Methods of study

Students were presented, in this question, with a list of study methods, which had been compiled from replies to a similar, but open-ended question in the pilot study diaries. They were asked to indicate all the study methods they used each day. The most popular method, when ranked by number of recorded instances of use, was 'reading over notes', and this was followed by the method 'reading from textbooks'. Ranked third, but considerably less often used, was 'writing notes neatly'. Next in order of recorded instances was 'making own notes from textbooks', with 'discussions with other students' coming fifth in rank order. The remaining three methods — 'drawing diagrams', 'reading handouts' and 'working from handouts' — were used relatively infrequently.

There was, in the main, a somewhat similar pattern in the methods of study over the five colleges. In Colleges I, II and V 'writing up notes neatly' was used by more than half of the students, whereas in colleges III and IV this was much less popular. College IV was outstanding in its use of the method 'discussions with other students' — 75% of students said they used this. College V students made least use of 'reading from textbooks', a very different picture from Colleges III and IV where more than 90% of students used this method.

There were no marked differences in study methods favoured by control or experimental group students.

SUMMARY

In conclusion, the general impression was that very little study was either required of students, or done by students in their own time. The Block timetables were full — almost every period occupied by a class on a specific subject from the syllabus. The evidence was of an emphasis, by teachers, on 'covering' the content of the course, and for students, of a somewhat passive recipient role, rather than an active, searching role in regard to learning. Many students relied heavily upon their notes, and a disturbingly high number, in the opinion of the researcher, rewrote notes neatly, a method which, if used without recourse to textbooks, is not only passive, but may compound any inaccuracies made at the time of the note-taking. It was interesting to link the emphasis upon notes in these diaries with the fact that several experimental group students felt 'lack of notes' to be a disadvantage of the experimental teaching method.

Study — whether required or done — reflects upon teacher as well as the taught. It can be presumed that the habit of study, or self-directed education, was not valued by teachers as so little appeared in the timetables. The study value may also not be inculcated in students if teachers do not look for the results of study, i.e. in papers or project work. It seemed unlikely that very much of that type of work was required of students when the average amount of time devoted to study was so very individual and so varied. The college where most study was recorded by students (College IV), was the one where the most variety of teaching methods was employed and one could speculate as to whether this led to more participation by students in their own learning, and to more being demanded of them in terms of self-directed learning, but that is a very tentative speculation, based as it is on such small numbers of students and on such a short and unusual period in their Block.

Study, insofar as the students in this sample were concerned, was the least popular method of teaching/learning, and was only very infrequently made use of in their daily work in Block.

16

Postscript

At a date suitable to each college, and usually at the beginning of the students' next theoretical component or Block, when the retention of learning tests were administered, the experimental group students completed a brief follow-up questionnaire.

It was interesting that, in spite of the passage of time, ranging from 16 weeks in College II to 29 weeks in the pilot college, the experimental group remained intact.

Looking back on it, all but one student viewed it positively.

TOTAL PATIENT CARE

Since their experience during the experiment, 23 (45%) students, from five of the six colleges, had had the opportunity to practise the method of giving nursing care used then, i.e. total patient care. The other 28 (55%) had not. Further details on this question were not available from pilot study questionnaires, but were available from the main study. For seven of those 23 who had given total patient care, this had been in only one ward, but for seven it had been in two different wards — medical, surgical and specialty wards were mentioned. Seven of the students had been 'specialling' a patient when carrying out total patient care.*

In three hospitals, those attached to Colleges III, IV and V, seven students said that they had worked on wards where sister organised the nursing by means of total patient care, but another six students, again from these same three colleges, had instigated this method of carrying out nursing care themselves, because they preferred to do it in this way:

> On night duty you were your own boss and you could run the ward and care for your patients as you felt.

---

* The term specialling is used to denote that one nurse is responsible for all the care required by one patient, usually someone who is very ill, and that the nurse is not responsible during that time for the care of any other patient.

Whenever I had been left in charge of the ward, I always preferred, if possible, that the same nurse did as much for the patient at the one time, rather than having different nurses coming backward and forward to carry out different procedures. I feel the patients appreciate total nursing care given by the one nurse at one session.

It is perhaps revealing of the system of nurse training that both the above students were one year and one month in training. However, it is also of interest that almost half of this small sample of students had worked in a situation where nursing care was organised with the emphasis on total patient care, rather than on the long dominant model of task assignment.

EFFECT OF EXPERIMENTAL COURSE UPON SUBSEQUENT NURSING

Mindful of the fact that the principal aim and function of nurse education is to prepare the student nurse for the work she must do, i.e. nursing, experimental group students were asked whether or not the experimental course had helped them in their nursing.

By a convincing majority, in all but one of the colleges, the course had helped. Forty (78%) students recorded a positive response. In the pilot college and Colleges IV and V of the main study this was a unanimous decision. Two of the senior students in College III, one student in College II and seven students in College I made a neutral response — the course had had no particular effect in their case. One student, again from College I, said that the course had created difficulties. Unfortunately she gave no clue as to these difficulties.

The response pattern to this question from students in College I was totally at variance with that of all other colleges, indeed the responses from students in College I had been quite different from the others on a number of occasions. There were two factors pertinent only to the students from this college which may have been of some influence on their opinions of the experimental method. Firstly, the experimental method had been introduced into their Block programme which, unlike the others, already included sessions when the students worked, mainly unsupervised, in the wards caring for two patients on whom they subsequently wrote up care studies. Secondly, College I students had no option to abstain from participation in the research.

From 39 of the 40 students who felt that the experimental course had helped them in their nursing, there was a wealth of comment available. Several had found it easier to learn and remember what they had been taught in college and use this knowledge in their work. They felt they understood their patients' conditions more fully. Some said they now took much more interest in their work, e.g. when a patient was admitted they would read up about his condition in case notes and books and could study more. Two students did mention that they felt there were some gaps in notes, and knowledge about certain diseases, which had not been dealt with in their course. Some mentioned that the course had increased their ability to obtain information directly from the patients:

> It has made me think about how to do things and why I do what I am doing and I don't have to keep asking about things because I can work them out for myself better.
> It has helped me to think more about how the patient's condition relates to his care — what he can do without causing pain, how long he needs total care and when he is able to do things for himself. Also to think more about why I am doing things and what the consequences will be if it is done properly or if he is given inadequate care.

As nurses, many found it had affected their attitudes and approach to patients, and had improved their personal standards of nursing care. They felt they now nursed more efficiently, understood the importance of the patient as a person, the advantages of planned and organised care and of performing the entire care required by a particular patient 'instead of doing one part and hoping someone else will do the rest'.

> It has helped in viewing the patient as a whole person more. Though that was always the intention, in the experiment I realised how often patients are left ignorant of what is happening in, and being done to their bodies. That there still is a lack of communication between nurses and medical staff as to how much the patient knows, who told them, and has anyone bothered, thinking someone else has.

The experimental method had also helped some students in dealing with patients' relatives, and others said that they gained in confidence. One student illustrated this in regard to being in charge of a surgical ward on night duty and being able to think back to similar situations in dealing with patients on the experimental course.

Two students' comments referred specifically to effects of their experience not just upon themselves but upon others:

My own personal standards are higher than they were and I hope it has rubbed off on some of the others.

This student had already found that some of the other nurses in the ward would not accept her way, nor the way they had been taught. A final percipient comment:

Although being part of the experiment has helped me in my nursing, on some occasions when certain procedures have been carried out in the wards I tend to feel I would like to change the system which I suppose could lead to problems.

PART 4

Summary and discussion

Whither nursing?

17

Summary and conclusions

This study was concerned with nurse education and training, in particular with the traditional college of nursing/hospital-based programme in Scotland, and the preparation of student nurses for the qualification of Registered General Nurse.

The question at the heart of the study was — how can integration of theory and practice in nursing be facilitated? The main aim of the study was the facilitation of such integration.

In pursuit of that aim, and of one possible answer to the question, an experiment was designed in which a planned programme of concurrent theory and directly relevant and supervised practice of nursing, i.e. of college and ward-based instruction, was experienced by student nurses randomly allocated to an experimental group. While their peers, in a control group, received teaching on the care of patients with gastrointestinal disease by entirely college-based methods, the experimental group both received teaching and carried out nursing care of such patients, during the hours allocated to that particular subject in their curriculum.

The main departures from the norm which were inherent in the experimental method of teaching/learning were:

(a) the cardinal importance of the students' learning needs in reaching the decision as to the nursing care they would carry out;

(b) the direct relevance of that care to the concurrent course of theoretical teaching;

(c) the students' freedom to concentrate only on the care of the chosen patients, i.e. they had no responsibility for the rest of the work of the ward during that time;

(d) their supervision by trained teachers — those who also participated in the theoretical input to the nursing course;

(e) the presence of the registered nurse teacher as part of the teaching team in the ward and at the patients' bedside;

(f) the identical role of the two grades of nurse teacher, throughout the period of the experiment, i.e. in both the ward-based and the college-based teaching;

(g) the type of communication and negotiation which took place between the teachers and the ward staff in finding appropriate patients for care by students in the experimental groups; (this communication was initiated by the researcher during the study)

(h) the element of control of the situation for the teacher when she arrived on the ward, in that she knew which patients her students would give care to, and could prepare her teaching plan beforehand;

(i) the flexi-time operated by the teachers — in that students and their teachers began work in the morning at the same time as the service staff, in order to avoid any necessity for ward staff to give them a separate report upon their patients. Instead they shared the morning report with the ward staff; and finally

(j) the approach to teaching and learning which followed the principles of active experiential learning. The intention was to help the students to *learn how to learn* from their daily work with patients. While planning their morning care with their teachers, students were encouraged to relate their background theoretical knowledge to their patient's condition and individual needs, and on returning to small group tutorials at the end of each period of practice, students were again encouraged to evaluate the care they had given; to look at similarities and differences in the care required and provided, in spite of perhaps identical Kardex diagnoses for various patients; and generally to examine facts previously learned in the context of the varied, and variable reality of patient care.

The research approach adopted was that of illuminative evaluation, an ecletic approach within which no one particular research method or technique need take precedence. For the evaluation of the experimental method of teaching/learning, *per se*, the pre-test, post-test, control group design (Campbell & Stanley, 1966) was chosen as most appropriate, and to this basic traditional design, a third stage was added, in which students' retention of learning was assessed, and also their opinions, in retrospect, about the teaching/learning method were obtained. It is the emphasis upon the opinions of those involved, i.e. the examination of any innovation *in context* which is the hallmark of the illuminative evaluation approach. Thus, pre-experiment opinions of students, ward trained staff and teachers as to aspects of the learning milieu in nursing were obtained, the day to day conduct of the experiment was documented, and the outcome measures included the opinions of all the participants as to the advantages and disadvantages of the innovation, their evaluation of whether the objectives of the experiment had been achieved, and also the test and essay scores of the students in both control and experimental groups.

Prior to the designing, implementation and evaluation of the experiment, a literature review and a short survey of four colleges of nursing were carried out.

The literature review examined first the system by means of which students learn to become nurses — the system of nurse education and training within which the problems of integration of theory and practice had arisen. As integration, the putting together of relevant parts to make a coherent and meaningful whole, was considered to be essentially an individual matter and a part of the active, ongoing process of learning, the next section of the literature review dealt with certain aspects of learning, in particular with active experiential learning and some of the ways in which students learn. The third and last part of the literature review dealt with the measurement and evaluation of learning and of educational programmes. In the survey, factual matters relating to the formal organisation of the colleges and the education and training programmes were ascertained, as were opinions of the teachers about the relationship of theory and practice in nursing.

The limitations of the research were mainly those inherent in educational research which is conducted within the 'untidy' reality of the classroom, as opposed to the much more controlled setting of the psychological learning laboratory, and compounded in this study by the fact that the teaching and learning also took place in the hospital wards where there were many additional uncontrolled variables. The patients, for example, were all different — the only common denominator was that they suffered from some form of disease of the gastrointestinal system; the experiment took place over a very short space of time, sample numbers were small, and the ubiquitous Hawthorne effect, as in any experiment, was a relevant interfering variable. However, against these and various other threats to the validity and the generalisability of the results of the study must be viewed the fact that the experiment was replicated, following its implementation in the pilot and first of the main study colleges, in four other main study colleges and their associated hospitals.

The findings and conclusions of the main study are summarised below. These were compiled from the contributions of an overall total of 119 student nurses, 224 ward trained staff and 72 teachers from the five main study colleges of nursing and their associated hospitals. These five colleges represented 26% of the 19 colleges of nursing and midwifery in Scotland.

THE MILIEU PRIOR TO THE INTERVENTION

In this study, all but one of the nurse teachers were found to occupy a generic role. A majority of the tutors taught most of the subjects in the General Nursing Council (Scotland) syllabus, and many had, in addition, overall administrative responsibilities for one or more intakes of students. Only 7% of the tutor sample said they taught often in the wards, 74% taught there rarely or not at all. All but one clinical teacher taught in a number of different wards and a variety of subjects.

Meetings, whether formal or informal, between college (teaching) staff and ward trained staff took place mainly at the instigation of the former, and were principally on matters directly connected with learners.

There was evidence of complete lack of communication between ward staff and teachers for more than one-third of the 224 ward staff, and 86% of the staff nurse respondents rarely or never met teaching staff of either grade.

70% of ward trained staff did not know whether or not a student nurse had had the relevant theoretical preparation for the work she was required to do in their particular ward. However, a majority of ward trained staff were involved in teaching student nurses while they were at work in their wards; indeed 97% of ward sisters considered they taught often or fairly often. Of the staff nurses, 89% said they taught often or fairly often, only two acknowledging that they never taught student nurses in the wards.

Against this background, and from all colleges, a total of 60% of the student sample recalled instances when their own ward nursing practice had differed from the taught method. Most examples quoted referred to procedures classified as technical nursing (Nuffield Job Analysis, 1953). Many also mentioned basic nursing and only 5% of the examples referred to affective nursing.

The following conclusions could be drawn from the comments: (a) respondents, many of whom were students only six months in training, had either failed to grasp principles of nursing care, or had not been taught principles; (b) certain nursing practices were clearly still in existence, in spite of many research findings to contraindicate their continued use; (c) there was evidence of careless, and at times dangerous practice — in particular in relation to nasogastric feeding of patients, the administration of medicines and the carrying out of surgical dressings, and (d) there was evidence of the existence of many rather than rare differences between theory and practice. Only 5% of the comments made referred to a patient, 95%

referred only to procedures. It is possible that this may have been a result of the phrasing of the question.

Integration of theory and practice was explained by some students as a college responsibility, a matter of appropriate timetabling or sequencing of theory and practice in their education and training programme, and by others as an individual responsibility of the student, to translate or put into practice what she had been taught.

Students considered their training programme lacked integration when (1) practice was not depicted realistically in the teaching, (2) theory was not followed by relevant ward practice, (3) ward staff appeared unaware of the students' stage of training and experience, and (4) there was evidence of conflicting values between college and ward. Theory and practice were considered well integrated when teaching, either in ward or college, was complementary and promoted students' understanding of patient needs, when specific links existed between the two environments, i.e. students went from college to the wards to carry out practice in relation to theory just taught. The senior students in the sample commented very favourably on their experience of study days, which they considered promoted integration of theory and practice by providing one day per week of theory which was directly relevant to current practice.

In the students' suggestions of measures to improve integration, there was a strong resemblance to some aspects of the experimental method, of which no student, at that time, had any foreknowledge.

Most of the ward teaching which students received while working on general medical and surgical wards was carried out by the staff nurses. Their contribution was consistently high, whether the teaching took the form of supervision and practical demonstration, or of short teaching and tutorial sessions. Other student nurses contributed almost as much to the former type of ward teaching as did the staff nurses, and considerably more than either the ward sister or the clinical teacher. The contribution of the registered nurse teacher was so small as to appear negligible. When the giving of tutorials was considered, the students in this sample considered the contribution of fellow student nurses to be less than that of the staff nurses, but very slightly more than that of the ward sister and the clinical teacher. Again, the contribution of the registered nurse teacher was negligible. 80% of the sample of students had never received supervision or practical demonstration on the wards from the registered tutor, and 91% had never received ward tutorials from her.

The students' perceptions appeared to be corroborated by the responses from ward staff and teachers to a similar question.

The methods of teaching used by the ward staff were predominantly the two above mentioned, namely teaching by supervised practice and demonstration, and by giving tutorials. 18% mentioned teaching by example, and only 6% teaching while giving the ward report.

In ranking a list of methods of teaching/learning — mainly college-based methods — in terms of their preferences, students showed clearly that their 'best-liked method' was the ward tutorial, and in answer to a different question, 77% of the sample said they learned most while working in the wards. From this, and some other indicators throughout the study results, it was concluded that ward-based teaching and learning was paramount for the students, yet the ward was the place where the contribution of the two grades of trained teachers was least, in terms of teaching, and that of the untrained teachers most. The registered nurse tutor, on whom most resources have been spent in teacher training, made almost no contribution, and the clinical teacher, whose *raison d'être* is ward teaching, made virtually the same contribution as the ward sister, and less than the staff nurses or other student nurses.

There was very strong support for the necessity for ward teaching of the student nurse while she was undergoing the practical component of her training, but a majority of ward trained staff and of teachers did not consider that the registered nurse teacher had a particular responsibility to provide such teaching, although she had a role to play.

When ward trained staff were asked who should take the main responsibility for ward teaching of students, 35% saw this as entirely the responsibility of the trained teachers, 35% considered it should be shared by education and service staff and 30% that it should be entirely a service staff responsibility. However, when those who had included the registered clinical teacher in their allocation of main responsibility for ward teaching were asked who should be responsible if no clinical teacher was available, very few indeed saw the registered nurse teacher as having any responsibility for ward teaching and 90% considered themselves, the untrained teachers, as solely responsible, in the absence of the clinical teacher.

Of the trained teachers, 71% considered the main responsibility for ward teaching should be either their own, or should be shared with service staff, but 29% considered it should be entirely the responsibility of the ward trained staff. Of those who had included the registered clinical teacher in their allocation of main responsibility for ward teaching, 62% considered that, in circumstances where no clinical teacher was available, only the ward trained staff (the untrained teachers) should bear responsibility.

According to 57% of the ward trained staff, the functions of the tutor and the clinical teacher, in regard to ward teaching, were different. In the main, the tutor was viewed as a theoretician and the clinical teacher as a practitioner of nursing, although a few of the ward staff added that the clinical teacher should link theory and practice. The trained teachers were evenly divided in their opinions, in that 50% considered functions of the two grades of teacher did differ, and 50% that they did not. Examples of differences given by the teachers were of their different course preparation, i.e. teacher training — whereby some tutors felt they were not prepared for the type of teaching required in the clinical area — and that the priorities of the two grades of teacher were very different, the clinical teacher having no, or very few teaching commitments other than in the ward, and the tutor having a considerable teaching commitment in the college.

Of the trained teachers, only the clinical teachers were asked if they considered functions differed between ward trained staff and themselves in regard to ward teaching, and 79% answered in the affirmative. 70% of ward trained staff also considered functions differed, and there was considerable agreement between clinical teachers and ward staff as to where the difference lay. Priorities were different — for the clinical teacher these lay with the student, for the ward staff with the patient; both groups saw the teacher training a distinct advantage, leading to differences in approach to teaching, and familiarity with various teaching methods for the clinical teacher. The latter's familiarity with the learners' needs, and links with the college of nursing were also quoted as examples leading to differences in function between the clinical teacher and the ward staff as teachers in the ward. There was a suggestion of the theoretician/practitioner division again, this time with the clinical teacher seeing herself as more able to teach theoretical aspects, than were the trained ward staff.

However, a clear majority of ward trained staff and of teachers considered the tutor *should* carry out ward teaching, although 8% of ward staff and 4% of teachers were unsure, and 1 tutor and 13 (6%) of the ward trained staff considered the tutor's place to be in the classroom and not in the ward.

FINDINGS AND CONCLUSIONS FROM THE POST–EXPERIMENT DATA

The experience of those involved with the experiment

Opinions as to what it was like to participate directly were available from 51 student nurses, 11 teachers and 58 ward staff.

The experiment was implemented in 7 hospitals and 33 wards and 91% of ward staff considered it caused no disruption to ward routine.

A fear, expressed before the commencement of the experiment by both teachers and students, that they would be required to carry out work on the wards other than had been previously arranged and which linked directly to their theoretical teaching, proved unfounded.

There was no difference in the role or function of the registered nurse teachers and the clinical teachers throughout the period of the experiment, and none considered they were required to do any work which was inconsistent with their appropriate role and function.

Those tutors who had not undergone a clinical teacher training course considered that their tutor training had prepared them adequately for the type of teaching required of them during the experiment. Four tutors who were also qualified clinical teachers considered that a clinical teaching course was essential preparation for the experimental teaching method, and that the tutor training course was not a suitable preparation for that type of teaching.

By a marked majority of opinion, effects of the experiment upon the ward staff were considered to be beneficial — workload was lighter, more time was available for other patients, and there was evidence that ward staff interest was stimulated. In two hospitals, both affected by ancillary staff strike action, two staff nurses feared experience might be taken away from ward student nurses.

84% of students felt that they had learned more as a result of the experimental method of teaching/learning, than they normally did using entirely college-based methods. However, pre-experiment opinions of students about a lack of supervision while working in the wards appeared corroborated by the post-experiment findings that several students were clearly unused to supervision. While 64% considered the supervision they received was 'just right', 30% of the students felt they required less supervision, in particular when they were giving basic care. All but one of that number were in their first year of training.

A majority of the ward staff and of the teachers were satisfied with the provision of supervision.

The most frequently expressed advantage of the experimental method was that of active, experiential learning. Terms used by students to describe their learning experience were 'finding out', 'talking over,' 'drawing together', 'seeing', 'doing' and 'associating'. All three groups of respondents considered it realistic learning. Students expressed approval of the less formal teaching methods and opportunities for more contact with tutors, and with the patients. Ward staff saw advantages for the students in their freedom from pressures and interruptions of ordinary ward work, and considered the opportunity for them to participate in total patient care was beneficial.

Teachers commented upon the opportunities for students 'to learn how to learn', in that they had more time to devote to one patient's care than was normal, and they received explicit encouragement to link theory and practice. Advantages for the teacher were in observing students at work, rectifying faults immediately, and co-ordinating theory and practice.

It was concluded that the advantages to the patients were considerable, both in the improved standard of care and in the fact that some were enabled to meet higher order needs, e.g. for self-actualisation and for self-esteem. It was also noted that, as a result of the experimental method, some students were alerted to the, at times, detrimental effects of their own well-intentioned efforts to 'care'.

No untoward effects were noted by any respondents upon the other patients in the wards.

One disadvantage mentioned by all three groups was that of lack of time. There were occasions when the two hours spent in the wards each morning were insufficient for the students to carry out the nursing care required by their patients and also to consult case notes and ward Kardex and then make their own notes. Teachers would also have preferred more time, both in the ward and in college in the seminar periods.

Some students felt a certain lack of security in that they had fewer notes than normal — a feeling intensified by an impression of the control group assiduously amassing notes in the classroom!

Ward staff felt that neither students nor the patient had continuity, in that students did not always return to nurse the same patient on a second morning. Students in one college developed an interesting coping strategy for this, which is discussed in the next chapter.

During the experiment students at no time went to the wards to carry out nursing procedures *per se*, but always to give individualised patient care. All but one of the students preferred total patient care to task assignment because they considered the former method (a) was better for the patient in that it provided possibilities for improved standards of care, (b) enhanced their own learning and increased their job satisfaction, and (c) facilitated teaching of junior nurses.

It was concluded that, for a majority of the students, the learning (affective) objectives (see p. 238) were attained insofar as these students were aware of the two different methods of organisation of patient care, i.e. patient assignment and task assignment, and valued the concept of individualised patient care. There was some evidence that the third of these affective objectives had been achieved by a small number of the students who had had the opportunity to practise total patient care in the period intervening between the experiment and their completion of the follow up questionnaire. 45% of the student sample had practised total patient care, and of that number half had done this on their own initiative.

There was a most encouragingly positive evaluation of the experimental method, not only from the experimental group students and their teachers, but also from the ward staff. The main objective, that of the facilitation of integration of theory and practice, received an entirely positive response from ward staff and teachers and from all but one of the students.

All but one of the experimental group teachers, and all but one of the control group teachers considered the method to be feasible within the present system of nurse education and training. One teacher was known to have already used the method, in slightly modified form, with more senior students, in circumstances unconnected with the research.

The experience of the control group teachers and students
There were control group students in four of the five colleges. A total of 56 students and eight teachers provided opinions as to their experience. The main difference as a result of the experiment was that class size was reduced, and lectures were concentrated into a shorter span of days than usual for that subject matter. Few found their experience disrupting. Those who did, complained of cramming, of intensive lectures and of feeling bored. Other comments were of the opposite vein, and evidenced Hawthorne effect, i.e. in increased interest as a result of the research.

Results of the tests and essays

Effectiveness of the course of instruction
Effective pairing of students in the experimental and control

groups, in terms of their knowledge of the subject matter of the course as measured by the objective test, was demonstrated prior to the experiment. There was a statistically significant gain score for students in both experimental and control groups from pre-test to post-test, and from pre-test to retention test (p < .001). It was concluded that both courses of instruction were effective.

The essays proved to be the more sensitive of the two measurements (i.e. objective test and essay type of test) in demonstrating forgetting between post-experiment and retention stages.

There was no statistically significant difference between students taught by the experimental method and those taught by the control method, nor was there any statistically significant difference at retention stage between students, in either group, for whom the intervening practical experience of nursing had been relevant to the subject matter of the experiment, and those for whom it had not.

There was a consistent trend for students from the experimental group to perform better than those in the control group on both tests and essays. This trend was extremely small at the post-experiment stage of immediate recall, but was more marked at the retention stage, though still not statistically significant.

Relationship between tests and essays and reliability of essay marking
Although the mean scores on the essays were, in every college, lower than the mean scores on the objective test, correlations between these two measures, when viewed across all colleges, were high, indicating a similar ordering of students on both measures. With regard to the marking of the essay scripts, there were significant differences between the means, and thus the marks awarded by the three neutral markers. There was very little difference however in the rank ordering of the students by the three markers.

Student nurses' study patterns
As a result of the findings in regard to study carried out during the admittedly abnormal period of the experiment, it was concluded that very little study was either required of the students in the sample, or done by these students in their own time.

Study, in so far as the pre-experiment sample of students were concerned, was the least popular method of teaching/learning, and for those of that number who took part in the experiment, either as experimental or control students, it was only infrequently made use of in their daily work in college.

18

Discussion and implications: some answers .... but more questions?

This research produced evidence, within the present system of nurse education and training, of various factors relevant to the problems of integration of theory and practice in nursing, but also produced evidence of one possible solution to certain of the problems. This was in the form of a method of teaching and learning about nursing in which theoretical teaching and relevant ward practice were combined in such a way as to provide an effective learning experience for the students concerned, enhanced job satisfaction for their teachers (both registered nurse teachers and registered clinical teachers shared an identical teaching role) and which had the support, approval and interest of the ward staff. What of the patients ... ?

TEACHING OF NURSING IN THE WARD — THE 'USE' OF PATIENTS

When the research experiment was in the early stages of planning, discussions between the researcher and colleagues in both education and service revealed that several feared there would be detrimental effects upon the patients directly involved. The view of the experimental method held by these nurses, as it transpired, was of a 'medical model' — of student nurses gathered around a patient's bedside, listening to a nurse teacher, i.e. passive learning, which 'used' patients. The reverse was true. Students learned by doing, by giving total care, as a result of which it *appeared* that the students became more aware of, more sensitive to the patients' individual needs, not just for basic physical care, but, for some patients, self-esteem needs, e.g. to feel important and of help to the students, and the need for a listening ear. Students not only commented upon this, but were found to spend time, of their own initiative, in trying to meet these needs for their patients. Given the situation of the experiment, students created opportunities to sit with patients, and 'just listen' because they felt that was the priority for the patient at the time. Several students, of their own accord, made a practice of returning each morning to see their patients of the day or days before, simply to talk with them.

There is a fairly widespread belief in nursing that students, and trained staff too, tend to busy themselves in tasks, and shy away from other than superficial and brief communication with their patients. This was not found to be the case for the students in the experimental groups, in that they showed sensitivity to patients' higher order needs as well as to those for basic care.

It is important in nursing that teachers, ward staff and students should be as aware of these higher order needs, as most are of the basic needs, and that these should be taught to and discussed with students, not only in relation to patients but to themselves and their co-workers. Yet it is the researcher's experience, as it is of other writers (Birch, 1972) that the behavioural sciences are not taught in nursing to a sufficient extent. Skills of communication, and such subjects as psychology and sociology are relevant in nursing, and should be taught in the classroom, and then the students helped to apply their theoretical knowledge to nursing, by their nurse teachers, in giving care to patients. However, if such subjects are introduced into the curriculum for the student nurses, there is then a concomitant responsibility for the profession to provide some form of continuing education in these matters for trained staff in post, lest the gap between theory and practice become even wider.

Students in the experimental groups were also sufficiently perceptive to note the possible effects of their greater involvement with patients as a result of providing total patient care. Altschul (1980) points out that while involvement may be good for patients, nurses need support so that they do not become over anxious at their possible inability to satisfy the patients' needs. A critical factor in such support is the understanding of the teacher, but also possession of background knowledge by the student, and the use of such teaching methods as involve small group discussion of these issues.

THE UNTRAINED TEACHERS

One of the very clear findings of this study was the extent to which the totally untrained in teaching were undertaking the ward teaching of the students in the sample. What were they teaching? The discrepancies between theory and practice noted in this, and in many other studies (Hunt, 1974; Bendall, 1975a; Jones, 1975) must, to a certain extent, have been connected with the fact that the staff nurses and student nurses did most of the ward teaching, yet these nurses are the most recently qualified, the most recent to emerge from the system of training, or, as is the case with the students, are still within that system. Is it peer group pressure to reject what has been taught in the college, is it lack of understanding of principles — as was seen at one point in this study — or is the teaching which emanates from the colleges unrealistic? There must be elements of this, and more, in the problem, but one of the effects of the evidence herein of the extent of the teaching done by staff nurses and student nurses must surely be that we begin, now, to teach student nurses to teach. This should be done from the very beginning of their education in nursing; done explicitly, not implicitly as often it is at present, and assessed regularly. For staff in post, workshops on teaching skills should be provided and their attendance encouraged. Preparation courses for future ward sisters should deal, in equal proportion, with the techniques of management and the techniques of teaching. The profession should debate the possibility, in the near future, of an identical preparation for the nurse teacher and the sister of a ward. The potential in terms of an interchangeable work force, and all that that would mean in promotion of understanding and communication is exciting to contemplate.

THE TEACHER IN HER COLLEGE

In this research, which took place in a quarter of the colleges of nursing in Scotland, and their associated hospitals, the trained teachers of nursing made little or no impact upon the teaching of nursing in the place where 77% of the students in the sample considered that they learned most about nursing, i.e. in the wards. Students had also voted their best liked method of teaching/learning, the ward tutorial; yet both grades of teacher, when compared with the ward sister, staff nurse and student nurses, contributed least of them all to the giving of ward tutorials. The implications, in terms of lost opportunities for teaching are considerable. Where learning is most likely to be seen as meaningful, where student motivation to learn is high, the untrained (in teaching skills) are left to make use of the most fertile ground. One cannot but wonder what might be achieved if the expert teacher was present in the wards to a greater extent, both to share in the teaching of students and also to support and guide the ward staff who are teaching. However, to wonder is not enough. In spite of improved teacher/learner ratios, in spite of the recommendations of the Briggs' Report (HMSO, 1972) and of the General Nursing Council (Scotland) (1976) that teachers of the practical activity of nursing should not be divorced from the wards, the trained teacher *is* divorced from the wards. This has been a fact in nursing for more than a century, and it seems no longer relevant or useful to deplore the fact — rather, it should be accepted, and the implications made explicit and dealt with constructively. This does not need legislation, or any major reshuffle, but can be done within the system of nurse education and training as it exists at present. The barriers to change, the difficulties, lie not in limited resources of finance or of manpower: 'the greatest impediments are found in the heart, not in the purse' (McGaghie, 1978, p. 89).

It was considered that there were a number of reasons apparent in the data from this research, which might in part explain the virtual seclusion of many nurse teachers in the colleges. Many of the more senior nurse teachers today are products of a time in nursing when the struggle was to procure set times when students were freed from responsibilities to give service, in order that they might attend lectures and study. The Block system was a hard-won achievement of many of those who today are reluctant to erode any of the time a student has away from the wards and in the college. It is interesting to reflect whether the crammed timetables of many Block programmes (noted in this and other studies) may be a relic of days when the sign of progress in nurse education was a student nurse, seated in a classroom, learning by listening, not learning by doing — the very passivity of her role as a learner seen as a welcome improvement to her general highly active role in the wards.

The teachers in this study, both tutors and clinical teachers, were generalists not specialists. Most tutors taught 'most of the subjects' in the General Nursing Council (Scotland) syllabus for general nursing. Many, in addition, were required to take administrative responsibility for one or more intakes of students. What are the effects of this formal organisation upon a newly qualified teacher of nurses who may wish to include ward teaching in her daily work? She is, as Birch (1972) pointed out, unlikely to be qualified, in terms of advanced knowledge, in any subject other than nursing, so she will inevitably have to spend much time and attention in preparing classes and in teaching subjects with which she is not wholly familiar or at ease. She enters a system where it is certainly not required, nor is it likely to be accepted practice to incur a responsibility for ward teaching — indeed she enters a system where there is already a teacher with a specific responsibility for ward teaching, namely the clinical teacher. The system is therefore such as to provide more disincentives than incentives for ward teaching by tutors, and in the vital early days of teaching a new tutor has less time available, and less power, as an inexperienced member of the teaching staff, to make or effect changes in the system in which the more experienced teachers are not themselves teaching in the wards. Her generic role as a registered nurse teacher — previously noted in this study and corroborated by the fact that it is still the exception rather than the rule to see a college advertisement for teachers with specialist knowledge — will combine with the above mentioned factors to make it difficult for her to avoid spending almost all of her time in the college of nursing. A pattern of work, once established, is more difficult to change, and as time goes by, a return to ward teaching becomes more problematic.

What might be the effects, if Directors of Nurse Education, together with their staff, agreed a policy which permitted all future posts to be advertised, and appointments made, on a specialist basis, as a first step towards facilitating an increased contribution to ward teaching by nurse tutors?

TWO GRADES OF TEACHER?

It appeared also from findings in this study that the creation of the clinical teacher grade had made it easier for the registered nurse teacher to opt out of ward teaching — surely an ironic and unforeseen result of the innovation of the late 1950s, intended as it was to improve links between theory and practice, college and ward. The teachers in this sample, who ranked various reasons why tutors did not teach in the wards, considered the fact that the clinical teacher was there, specifically to carry out ward teaching, to be the *most* likely reason for the non-appearance of many tutors on the wards. They considered it a more likely reason than pressure of college commitments, or even the possibility that the tutor had gradually lost contact with ward work.

In view of this finding, it is recommended that in Scotland, further research should be done, in order to decide whether the continuation of two grades of nurse teacher is of value, or counterproductive to the General Nursing Council's stated aim to have tutors assume some responsibility for ward teaching. The question must be raised — is one of the answers to the problem of integration of theory and practice simply to have one grade of teacher — no 'middleman' between the classroom lesson and the practical application of that lesson?

WARD TEACHING — WHOSE ROLE?

There was evidence of both lack of understanding of the role or function of the tutor as a ward teacher, and of a lack of communication generally between education and service staff in this study. A majority of ward staff considered that, in a situation where no clinical teacher was available, they held the responsibility for teaching students in the ward, and not the tutor. Although most felt the tutor had some role to play in ward teaching, a minority were not at all sure of this or considered the tutor's place to be in the classroom not the ward. The implications of the above points are far-reaching and serious. Firstly, for the student, they mean that any ward teaching she is given, or practice she carries out, is unlikely to be planned in accord with her learning needs, or with her current knowledge-base in mind — in fact teaching and practice must proceed on an *ad hoc* basis. That this may well be so is implied in the way in which the experimental method of teaching/learning was seen, in all but one college, as a novel development and in the interest shown and the questions asked by the ward staff involved in the choice of suitable patients for the students, with the researcher and the teachers.

Secondly, implications for future recruitment to nurse teaching must be considered. As a factor in improving communications, current efforts to bring ward staff to the college of nursing are helpful, but limited in usefulness because such visits tend to be of passive observation, rather than of active involvement in teaching. The latter was found, for this study, to be carried out by very few indeed of the ward staff. The answer to more effective communication must lie, principally, in an increase of traffic in the other direction, because of the important implications of a nurse teacher role model who is not in the wards, but, as one ward sister respondent said: 'in the peace and calm of the classroom'. Potential teachers, seeing the current situation, may be drawn to a career which they see as quite apart from nursing practice, and pursue it because they wish to leave the practical areas altogether — thus maintaining the *status quo* in teaching or alternatively, other potential recruits may be lost because they cannot see how teaching and practice of nursing can be combined.

In view of all of the above, is it therefore surprising to find the main emphasis, in the current suggestions for improvements in nurse education, not upon tutors leaving college to teach in the wards, nor upon the Block students leaving college in order to make links between teaching and practice (although there are pockets of such innovations), but upon improved ordering of theory and practice, upon modular programmes, upon preserving if not increasing the proportion of the students' training spent in the classroom, *vis-à-vis* the time spent in practice?

Such improvements, in particular the modular programmes, while important, are not of themselves adequate to improve integration of theory and practice in nursing. While the formal organisation of work in the colleges is unaltered, while the generic role of both grades of teacher continues, while the whole accent in teaching is on the didactic, rather than on involving the student in active, participative forms of teaching and learning, many of the problems of integration will remain largely unsolved. It is therefore recommended, that following upon the first step of the appointment of specialist nurse teachers, all newcomers to teaching be enabled, and expected to undertake responsibilities for ward teaching in which active experiential learning is the predominant method of teaching and learning for the subject of nursing. It is suggested, on the evidence of this research, that this be done, for the present, with students who are in Block, and not with students who are on the ward staff. By taking Block students, i.e. working within the system as it exists, teachers have the best possibilities for the carrying out of planned and co-ordinated teaching of theory and practice in nursing.

A CONTROVERSIAL VIEW OF RATIOS

Although ratios of trained staff to learners on the wards in the hospitals in this study were never less than 1 : 2, and in many general wards were 1 : 1, nonetheless, the considerable fluctuations in the numbers of learners, and their short stay in each ward, give problems which mitigate against either teachers or ward staff giving regular and planned teaching to the constant flow of new learners.

Ratios of teachers to students on the other hand merit closer examination. These may not be what they seem. Figures quoted in the General Nursing Council (Scotland) Reports refer to all teaching staff and ratios are quoted (excluding the Directors and Assistant Directors of Education) in relation to learners in training, i.e. a period of 144 weeks. Results in this research, and borne out by the literature, show that on the whole very little classroom teaching is done by clinical teachers and very little ward teaching is done by registered nurse teachers. If therefore one considers (1) that many tutors are working with students only while they are in Block, and (2) that only approximately one sixth of the students' time is spent in Block throughout training, then one may be justified in looking at the ratios a little differently.

General Nursing Council (Scotland) figures for 1978 stated that there were 519 teaching staff, giving a ratio of 1 : 19. 268, or approximately half of the total teaching staff were registered nurse tutors, giving a ratio of 1 : 38, but if these tutors are primarily in the college and only one-sixth of the students' time is spent there, then one can postulate a ratio of 1 : 6 while the student is in college or Block. If one were to abandon, for an experimental period, the deployment of the clinical teacher in teaching learners who were part of the ward staff, and, as was done in the research experiment, concentrate her activities upon the teaching and supervision of students attending wards from college, this would permit the inclusion of both grades of teacher in the ratio — the result, a ratio of 1 : 3* — much more favourable than appeared at first sight. It would concentrate skilled resources where and when the student is potentially most able to benefit, i.e. free from ward work and responsibilities and currently receiving theoretical teaching, i.e. she is a student not only in name but in reality, and the priority is her teaching and her learning. It is suggested therefore that the method used in the experiment is a reasonable and feasible alternative to the present deployment of teachers of nursing, and that it may eradicate some of the present problems of ward teaching and of integration, by increasing communication between college and ward staff, fostering closer working relationships between tutors and clinical teachers, and involving students in active learning at a time when they have no other responsibilities in their work other than to their own learning.

KNOWLEDGE WHICH IS CONTEXTUAL AND RELATIVE

An important and overdue change in nursing education towards more involvement of students in their own learning would also be facilitated by the method above proposed. Active, rather than passive learning would be predominant, and there would be opportunities for much more participation between student and teacher in the learning process. It is essential that the type of thinking which is basic to discovery learning, to problem-solving in relation to the needs of individual patients, be fostered and developed in students

---

* Although the 1980 General Nursing Council (Scotland) report showed a slightly poorer ratio of teachers to learners (1 : 22.7), the comparable ratio, calculated as above, remains favourable, i.e. 1 : 4.

of nursing, simply because so much of the knowledge required in nursing is contextual and relative, rather than, to use Perry's term (1975) 'a collection of discrete rightnesses'. (This matter is discussed in Chapter 3, p. 47).

There were clues within the research that there was a lack of appreciation by students of the relative nature of nursing. Also the fact that so many saw classroom teaching as helpful, yet not relating well to practice may indicate that, as Wong (1979) pointed out, they fail to see the necessity to transfer knowledge from classroom to work, or that classroom learning is 'learning from the neck up' (Rogers, 1969). A disturbing finding was of how little study was required of and done by students in the sample, and also the finding that they did not like any form of study; in particular they disliked self-directed study. Such attitudes, though understandable, in that most students enjoy 'spoonfeeding', are of course of concern when the students' task in learning to nurse is integrational. Most of the behaviour required of the nurse at work is too complex to specify precisely, and thus she must transfer what she has learned to the performance of behaviour it has not been possible to analyse. To do this successfully she must be able to think things out for herself. At work on the wards she is expected to make decisions, to apply principles, yet how can she do this if she is not actively involved in the process of learning, if the predominant teaching methods in the college are directed to passive reception on the learners' part, to safely covering the syllabus on the teachers' part?

THE TEACHER AS FACILITATOR

The experimental method of learning was based upon the principles of active experiential and meaningful learning put forward by C. Rogers, Ausubel and Maslow. Students were placed in direct confrontation with nursing care and problems which were a part of normal daily nursing work. This type of approach, including as it did the participation of students and teachers in a seminar following each period of ward practice, has been documented as both exacting and stimulating for the teacher, as well as for the student, but, it is pointed out, the quality of the instructors is decisive (World Health Organisation, 1966).

The role of the teacher in such teaching is quite different from her role as 'lecturer' or 'demonstrator'. It is the role of the 'facilitator' described by both Rogers and Maslow above referred to, enabling students to grow towards their full potential. It is a difficult role, one which many teachers are afraid of as they have less control over what will occur in the classroom. In the reluctance of many to embark on such teaching may be seen one of the problems at the root of ward teaching for tutors. There is no doubt that the teacher must be prepared for such a role in her teacher training course. Teachers in the experiment found their role both exacting and stimulating, and they were divided in their opinions as to whether they had received adequate preparation for this in their own trainings. It may be that the content, and teaching methods in which experience is gained in these courses, should be examined by those concerned in the profession, and that determined efforts be made both to secure able candidates for the more difficult role of the facilitator and to provide an appropriate and adequate preparatory course, for there is no doubt that the more relevant role for the teacher of nurses is that of the facilitator rather than the spoon-feeder.

NO ONE 'BEST' METHOD OF TEACHING

Although the emphasis in this discussion has been upon the benefits of the active learning of the experimental method, it is stressed that variety of methods of teaching is important. Only in this way, can the wide individual differences among students be catered for; can all be enabled to learn. While some members of a class of student nurses are learning how to nurse in the method described and carried out in the experiment, others in the same class could be employed in other forms of active learning. There should be much more encouragement of study, and expectation, by teachers, of evidence of study by their students. Clearly, from the commencement of training, students would require to be introduced to active, participative forms of learning.

Teachers will always debate what is the best use of their own, and the students' time while in the Block, and there is little doubt that some of the methods herein advocated are more time-consuming than the lecture method, with its attractive air of economy, in that an entire class of students can be addressed in a period which can, if desired, be packed with factual information. While lectures will always have some place in nursing education, are they the medium of choice for teachers of *nursing* when teaching the subject of *nursing*? That is doubtful.

If experts in the fields of biological sciences and behavioural sciences were employed to teach theoretical aspects of these subjects, would not the teacher of nursing be freed for the more exacting, more time-consuming but surely more relevant task of helping the student to apply that knowledge in the care of patients? Even more importantly, would the nurse teacher then go to the wards, there very deliberately to teach the student to learn how to learn from the richness of experience available to her in the wards, or indeed the homes of the patients. There is potential is such a system for continuity of care in that students might be able to follow patients from hospital to home, to achieve their heretofore problematic community care experience in a much more personal and relevant way than occurs in nurse training at present. The use of computer records of student nurse experience would make straightforward the calculation of experience of community work for individual students, so that any necessary arrangements could be made to ensure adequate amounts of such experience. Should this be the subject of a future research experiment in nursing?

It would also be most interesting to see research done on the ways in which students learn about nursing, on the learning processes they adopt in whatever studying they do. There have been three recent studies on learning environment in nursing (Fretwell, 1979, Ogier, 1980 and Orton 1980), but, to the researcher's knowledge, no work akin to that of Marton & Säljö, (1976; 1976a) or of Pask (1976) on styles and strategies of learning, has been carried out with student nurses.

It would also be of interest to see the present research replicated, perhaps with students at different stages of training, or preparing for registration on other than the General Register, and also with students in the new modular programmes.

SUMMARY

In summary, there were four main recommendations in the substance of the above discussion. These were based upon evidence in the pre-experiment qualitative data, upon the strong endorsement of the experiment by student nurses, ward staff and teachers, upon its reported benefits to the patients, and notwithstanding the lack of a statistically significant result on the test scores — which latter result was considered to be not unrealistic in view of the brevity of the intervention. These recommendations were:

(1) that teachers of nursing teach nursing where nursing is carried out — that they do this particularly with students who are temporarily freed from the pressures of responsibility for providing service, i.e. are in Block, but who remain within the apprenticeship system of nurse education and training;

(2) that teaching methods which actively involve the student in her own learning become the rule rather than the exception within a richer variety of teaching methods used in nursing curricula;

(3) that attention be directed to the effects, within nurse education and training, of the existence of two grades of nurse teacher;

(4) as a matter of urgency, that attention be given to teaching ward staff and student nurses to teach.

CONCLUSION

This research was about nursing — the experiment was about learning to nurse; learning to establish positive links between what was taught and what was practised in nursing; learning to integrate theory and practice. There are many facets to integration of theory and practice in nursing and many ways in which it can be facilitated or hindered, but ultimately, the actual achievement of integration is a matter for the individual student. It is a part of the active, dynamic process of individual learning, and as such, it neither can be measured, nor appropriately expected or sought, as a result of the very brief learning experience of the experimental group students. Gagné (1971) states:

> One does not 'teach the student to think' by means of a single course in thinking. Instead, if he is properly challenged, he continues to become a better thinker all his life long. (p 522)

One does not teach student nurses to integrate theory and practice by means of a single course in integrating, but, properly challenged . . . ?

> It brought out all the simple little things that made everything fit in.

(Student in the experimental group)

References

Chapter 1

Bendall E 1977 The future of British nurse education. Journal of Advanced Nursing 2 (2): 171–181

General Nursing Council for Scotland 1973 Syllabuses for nursing (Reprint). General Nursing Council for Scotland, Edinburgh

General Nursing Council for Scotland 1978 Schemes of training for the register of nurses. Document issued to the Area Nurse Training Committees and Colleges of Nursing and Midwifery in Scotland. General Nursing Council for Scotland, Edinburgh

Henderson V 1966 The nature of nursing. MacMillan, New York

Jackson B, Marsden D 1969 Education and the working class. Penguin, Middlesex

Roper N 1976 Clinical experience in nurse education. Churchill Livingstone, Edinburgh

Whitty G, Young M (eds) 1976 Explorations in the politics of school knowledge. Studies in Education Ltd., Mafferton, England

Chapter 2

Abdel-Al H 1975 Relating education to practice within a nursing context. Unpublished PhD thesis, University of Edinburgh

Altschul A 1978 A measure of education. Unpublished paper given at annual conference of Royal College of Nursing Association of Nursing Education, London

Balme H 1937 A criticism of nursing education. Oxford University Press, London

Baly M E 1973 Nursing and social change. Heinemann Medical, London

Bendall E 1971 The learning process in student nurses. Nursing Times Occasional Papers 1 and 2 67(43 and 44)

Bendall E 1973 The relationship between recall and application of learning in trainee nurses. Unpublished PhD thesis, University of London

Birch J A 1972 An investigation into the cause of wastage during nurse training. Unpublished MEd thesis, University of Newcastle upon Tyne

Birch J A 1978 Anxiety in nurse education. Unpublished PhD thesis, University of Newcastle upon Tyne

Brotherstone J 1960 Research mindedness and the health professions. In: Learning to investigate nursing problems. Report of an International Seminar on Research in Nursing, Delhi, India. International Council of Nurses and Florence Nightingale International Foundation, London

Brown E L 1948 Nursing for the future. Russell Sage Foundation, New York

Carter G B 1939 A new deal for nurses. Gollancz, London

Dalton B M 1969 Withdrawal from training of RNMS student nurses. Nursing Times Occasional Paper 2 65(3)

Dodd A P 1974 Towards an understanding of nursing. Unpublished PhD thesis, University of London

Edwards M M 1962 Some nursing reports. (Nursing Times Reprint) McMillan & Co., London

Ferguson A C 1976 De-schooling nurses. Nursing Times 72(48): 1864

General Nursing Council for Scotland 1976 Annual report. General Nursing Council for Scotland, Edinburgh

General Nursing Council for Scotland 1978 Schemes of training for the register of Nurses. Document issued to the Area Nurse Training Committees and Colleges of Nursing and Midwifery in Scotland. General Nursing Council for Scotland, Edinburgh

Goldmark J 1923 Nursing and nursing education in the United States. Report of the Committee on the Study of Nursing Eucation, New York

Gott M 1979 Student nurses: introductory course preparation and work world expectations. International Journal of Nursing Studies 16(4): 307–317

Halliburton J C 1976 Internal evaluation of an experimental dacum curriculum in a diploma school of nursing. Unpublished EdD thesis, Boston University School of Education

Harrison J, Saunders M E, Sims A 1977 Integrating theory and practice in modular schemes for basic nurse education. Journal of Advanced Nursing 2(5): 503–519

HMSO 1972 Report of the Committee on Nursing (The Briggs Report) Cmnd 5115. HMSO, London

Hoûe E 1978 Aspects of nursing education in the United Kingdom: A study with particular reference to innovation, change, evaluation and research. Unpublished report prepared for Nursing Research Unit, University of Edinburgh

Hughes E C, Thorne B, De Boggis A M, Gurin A, Williams D 1973 Education for the professions of medicine, law, theology and social welfare. McGraw Hill, New York

Hunt J M 1971 The teaching and practice of basic nursing procedures in three hospitals. Unpublished MPhil thesis, University of Surrey

Hutchings M 1981 A critique of Bendall's So you passed, Nurse. Journal of Advanced Nursing 6(5): 405–408

Jamieson E M, Sewall M F 1954 Trends in nursing history. Saunders, London

Jones D C 1975 Food for thought. Royal College of Nursing, London

Kelly E M 1980 Bolton's introductory course. Nursing Times 76(5): 213–214

Kirkwood L 1979 The clinical teacher. Nursing Times Occasional Paper 75(12)

Kramer M 1974 Reality shock. C V Mosby, St Louis

Lamond N 1970 The Registered Nurses' view of general student nurse education. Unpublished MLitt thesis, Aberdeen University

Lancet 1932 The report of the Lancet Commission on nursing. The Lancet, London

Macguire J 1969 Threshold to nursing. Occasional Papers on Social Administration, No.30. Bell, London

Martin J L 1973 The scope for learning. Nursing Times Occasional Paper 69(29)

Nuffield Provincial Hospitals Trust 1953 Work of nurses in hospital wards. Report of a Job Analysis. Nuffield Provincial Hospitals Trust, London

Robertson C M 1979 The development of clinical teaching. Nursing Times 75(25): 1063–1064

Roper N 1976 Clinical experience in nurse education. Churchill Livingstone, Edinburgh

Royal College of Nursing and National Council of Nurses of the United Kingdom 1964 A reform of nursing education — first report of a special committee on nurse education. Royal College of Nursing and National Council of Nurses of the United Kingdom, London

Scott Wright M 1961 A study of the performance of student nurses in relation to a new method of training with special reference to the evaluation of an experimental course of basic nursing education being conducted in Scotland. Unpublished PhD thesis, University of Edinburgh

Scottish Home and Health Department 1963 Experimental nurse training at Glasgow Royal Infirmary. HMSO, Edinburgh

Strohmann R 1977 Improving student clinical experiences. Nursing Outlook 25(7): 460–462

Taylor J 1979 The opinions and expectations of the staff and students involved in an experimental introductory course for student nurses. Unpublished dissertation towards the Award in Advanced Study in Technical Education of the University of Manchester

Chapter 3

Ausubel D P 1968 Educational psychology: a cognitive view. Holt, Rinehart and Winston, New York

Ausubel D P, Robinson F G 1969 School learning: an introduction to educational psychology. Holt, Rinehart and Winston, New York

Ausubel D P 1975 Cognitive structure and transfer. In: Entwistle N J, Hounsell D J (eds) How students learn. Institute for Research and Development in Post-compulsory Education, University of Lancaster

Balson D M 1969 The effectiveness of programmed learning in promoting transfer in a training situation. Programmed Learning and Educational Technology 6: 159–163

Bendall E 1973 The relationship between recall and application of learning in trainee nurses. Unpublished PhD thesis, University of London

Bendall E 1975 Learning. In: Raybould E (ed) A guide for teachers of nurses. Blackwell Scientific Publications, Edinburgh

Bigge M L 1971 Learning theories for teachers. Harper and Row, New York

Bloom B S (ed) 1956 Taxonomy of educational objectives, Book 1 Cognitive domain, paperback edn. Longman, London

Boydell T 1976 Experiential learning. Department of Adult Education, University of Manchester

Cronbach L J 1977 Educational psychology, 3rd edn. Harcourt, Brace, Jovanovich, New York

Entwistle N, Hounsell D 1975 How students learn: implications for teaching in higher education. In: Entwistle N, Hounsell D J (eds) How students learn. Institute for Research and Development in Post-compulsory Education, University of Lancaster

Fretwell J E 1978 Socialisation of nurses: teaching and learning in hospital wards. Unpublished PhD thesis, University of Warwick

Gagné R M 1970 The conditions of learning, 2nd edn. Holt, Rinehart and Winston, New York

Gagné R M 1971 Instruction based on research in learning. Engineering Education 61: 519–523

Glaser R 1962 Psychology and industrial technology. In: Glaser R (ed) Training, research and education. Wiley, New York

Goodwin W L, Klausmeier H J 1975 Facilitating student learning. Harper and Row, New York

Green J L 1974 The relationship between membership in a curricular preference typology and selected performance outcomes. Unpublished PhD thesis, University of California

Guimei M K 1977 Effectiveness of a programmed instruction module on oral contraceptives. Nursing Research 26(6): 452–455

Harding L 1979 The role of the teacher in the clinical field. In: Hinchliff S M (ed) Teaching clinical nursing. Churchill Livingstone, Edinburgh

Heath J 1979 Tomorrow's approach to learning. Nursing Mirror 149(6): 22–23

Henderson V 1966 The nature of nursing. MacMillan, New York

Hills P 1979 Teaching and learning as a communication process. Croom Helm, London

Hockey L 1980 Challenges for nursing. Nursing Times 76(21): 908–911

Hunt J M 1971 The teaching and practice of basic nursing procedures in three hospitals. Unpublished M. Phil thesis, University of Surrey

Hutty H E 1965 Student nurses: first year problems. Unpublished MSc thesis, University of Manchester

Isaacs B J, Hull E J 1975 Programmed learning. In: Raybould E (ed) A guide for teachers of nurses. Blackwell Scientific Publications, Edinburgh

Judd C H 1939 Educational psychology. Allen & Unwin, London

Kulhavy R W, Anderson R C 1972 Delay retention effect with multiple choice tests. Journal of Educational Psychology 63: 505–512

McKeachie W J 1975 The decline and fall of the laws of learning. In: Entwistle N J, Hounsell D J (eds) How students learn. Institute for Research and Development in Post-compulsory Education, University of Lancaster

MacMillan P 1980 Paid to think? Nursing Times 75(3): 101

Marton F 1975 What does it take to learn? In: Entwistle N J, Hounsell D J (eds) How students learn. Institute for Research and Development in Post-compulsory Education, University of Lancaster

Marton F, Säljö R 1976 On qualitative differences in learning: I Outcome and process. The British Journal of Educational Psychology 46(Part 1): 4–11

Marton F, Säljö R 1976a On qualitative differences in learning: II Outcome as a function of the learner's conception of the task. The British Journal of Educational Psychology 46(Part 2): 115–127

Maslow A H 1968 Some educational implications of the humanistic psychologies. Harvard Educational Review 38(4): 685–696

Maslow A H 1974 What is a Taoistic teacher? In: Rubin L J (ed) Facts and feelings in the classroom. Ward Lock Educational, London

Maslow A H 1975 Goals and Implications of humanistic education. In: Entwistle N J, Hounsell D J (eds) How students learn. Institute for Research and Development in Post-compulsory Education, University of Lancaster

Miller C M L, Parlett M 1974 Up to the mark. Society for Research into Higher Education, London

Munn N L 1966 Psychology, 5th edn. Houghton Mifflin, Boston

Ogier M E 1980 A study of the ward sister's leadership style and verbal interaction with nurse learners. Unpublished PhD thesis, University of London

Orton H D 1980 Ward learning climate and student nurse response. Unpublished MPhil thesis, Sheffield City Polytechnic

Pask G 1969 Strategy, competence and conversation as determinants of learning. Programmed Learning 6(4): 250–267

Pask G 1976 Conversational techniques in the study and practice of education. British Journal of Educational Psychology 46(Part1): 12–25

Pask G, Scott B E 1972 Learning strategies and individual competence. International Journal of Man machine Studies 4: 217–253

Perry W G Jr. 1975 Intellectual and ethical development in the college years. In: Entwistle N J, Hounsell D J (eds) How students learn. Institute for Research and Development in Post-compulsory Education, University of Lancaster

Rogers C 1969 Freedom to learn. C N Merril, Columbus, Ohio

Roueche J E 1975 New learning principles. In: Entwistle N J, Hounsell D J (eds) How students learn. Institute for Research and Development in Post-compulsory Education, University of Lancaster

Silvey H M 1951 Student reaction to the objective and essay test. School and Society 73: 377–378

Sturges P T 1972 Information delay and retention: effect of information in feedback and tests. Journal of Educational Psychology 63: 32–43

Taylor J 1979 The opinions and expectations of the staff and students involved in an experimental introductory course for student nurses. Unpublished dissertation towards the Award in Advanced Study in Technical Education of the University of Manchester

Thorndike E L 1924 Mental discipline in high school studies. Journal of Educational Psychology 15: 1–22 and 83–98

Vickers G 1973 Educational criteria for times of change. Journal of Curriculum Studies 5: 13–24

Wong J 1979 The inability to transfer classroom learning to clinical nursing practice: a learning problem and its remedial plan. Journal of Advanced Nursing 4(2) 161–168

Chapter 4

Allen M 1977 Evaluation of educational programmes in nursing. World Health Organisation, Geneva

Allen M, Reidy M 1971 Learning to nurse: the first five years of the Ryerson nursing program. Registered Nurses' Association of Ontario, Toronto

Beck F 1958 Basic nursing education. International Council of Nurses, London

Bendall E 1973 The relationship between recall and application of learning in trainee nurses. Unpublished PhD thesis, University of London

Birch J A 1975 To nurse or not to nurse. Royal College of Nursing and National Council of Nurses of the U.K., London

Cooper K 1976 Curriculum evaluation definitions and boundaries. In: Tawney D (ed) Curriculum evaluation today: trends and implications. (Schools Council Research Studies) Macmillan Education, London

Cox C 1979 Unpublished paper given at Community Outlook Conference, York University and reported in Nursing Times (Community Outlook Supplement) 75 (45): 348

Cronbach L J 1977 Educational psychology, 3rd edn. Harcourt, Brace, Jovanovich, New York

Dagsland H 1965 Lederskap i skolen. Norsk Sykepleierforlund, Oslo

De Landsheere V 1979 On defining educational objectives. Evaluation in Education Vol. I

Du Bois P H 1966 A test-dominated society: China 1115 BC–AD 1905. In: Anastasi A (ed) Testing problems in perspective. American Council on Education, Washington, D. C.

Ebel R L 1979 Essentials of educational measurement 3rd edn. Prentice Hall, Englewood Cliffs, N. J.

Finlayson D S 1951 The reliability of the marking of essays. The British Journal of Educational Psychology XXI: 126–134

Glaser R 1963 Instructional technology and the measurement of learning outcomes–some questions. American Psychologist 18: 519–521

Goodwin W L, Klausmeier H J 1975 Facilitating student learning. Harper and Row, New York

Green J L, Stone J C 1977 Curriculum evaluation, theory and practice. Springer Publishing, New York

Haley A 1977 Roots. Hutchinson, London

Harlen W 1976 Change and development in evaluation strategy. In: Tawney D (ed) Curriculum evaluation today: trends and implications. (Schools Council Research Studies) Macmillan Education, London

Hartog P, Rhodes E C 1936 The marks of examiners. MacMillan, London

Hartog P, Rhodes E C 1936a An examination of examinations. MacMillan, London

Hauf B J 1975 An evaluative study of a non-traditional field placement for community health nursing students. Unpublished EdD thesis, University of Montana

Hopkins R, Wright V 1978 The best way to lecture in rheumatology. Nursing Times 74 (51): 2115–2116

House V 1977 Evaluation research: the need for multiple criteria. Journal of Advanced Nursing 2 (1): 15–20

House V 1977a Survival of the fittest: a summary of an attempt to evaluate experimental schemes of nurse training. Journal of Advanced Nursing 2 (2): 157–170

Hunt J M 1974 The teaching and practice of surgical dressings in three hospitals. Royal College of Nursing, London

Joint Board of Clinical Nursing Studies 1978 Course evaluation package. Occasional Publication 2, Joint Board of Clinical Nursing Studies, London

Katz F M 1978 Guidelines for evaluating a training programme for health personnel. World Health Organisation, Geneva

Lamond N 1974 Becoming a nurse. Royal College of Nursing and National Council of Nurses of the U.K., London

Logan W W, Grosvenor P A 1970 Students' reactions to an educational programme: I. Nursing Times Occasional Papers 66(9) 33–35

Logan W W, Grosvenor P A 1970 Students' reactions to an educational programme: II. Nursing Times Occasional Papers 66 (10): 37–39

Mager R F 1962 Preparing instructional objectives. Fearon Publishers, Belmont, curriculum development in medical education. (Public Health Papers No. 68) World Health Organisation, Geneva

Mager R F 1962 Preparing instructional objectives. Fearon Publishers Belmont, California

Mehrens W A, Lehmann I J 1978 Measurement and evaluation in education and psychology, 2nd edn. Holt, Rinehart & Winston, New York

Meleis A I, Benner P 1975 Process or product evaluation. Nursing Outlook 23 (5): 303–307

Miller C M L, Parlett M 1974 Up to the mark. Society for Research into Higher Education, London

Nisbet J D 1974 Educational research, the state of the art, Cited by McDonald B 1976 Evaluation and the control of education. In: Tawney D (ed) Curriculum evaluation today: trends and implications. MacMillan Education, London

Nisbet J D, Entwistle N J 1973 The psychologists' contribution to educational research. In: Taylor W (ed) Research perspectives in education. Routledge and Kegan Paul, London

Ogundeyin W M 1980 Effectiveness of self instructional units in post-basic nursing education. Journal of Advanced Nursing 5 (2) 169–178

Overton P, Stinson S M 1977 Programme evaluation in health services: the use of experimental designs. Journal of Advanced Nursing 2 (2): 137–146

Pensivy B A 1977 Traditional versus individualised nursing instruction. Journal of Nurse Education 16 (2): 14–23

Peters R S, White J P 1973 The philosophers' contribution to educational research. In: Taylor W (ed) Research perspectives in education. Routledge and Kegan Paul, London

Pilliner A E G 1973 Experiment in educational research. (Block 5 of Educational studies: a third level course, methods of educational enquiry) Open University Press, Bletchley

Pilliner A E G 1977 Report to the Vice Chancellor of Tribhuvan University and to the British Council University Examinations in Nepal. Internal publication by The Godfrey Thomson Unit for Academic Assessment, The Centre for Research in the Educational Sciences, University of Edinburgh

Pomeranz R 1973 The lady apprentices. Occasional Paper on Social Administration No. 51. Bell, London

Popham J 1978 Criterion referenced measurement. Prentice Hall, New Jersey

Rowntree D 1974 Educational technology in curriculum development. Harper and Row, London

Scott Wright M 1961 A study of the performance of student nurses in relation to a new method of training with special reference to the evaluation of an experimental course of basic nursing education being conducted in Scotland. Unpublished PhD thesis, University of Edinburgh

Scriven M 1967 The methodology of evaluation. In: Tyler R W, Gagné R M, Scriven M (eds) Perspectives of curriculum evaluation. Rand McNally, Chicago

Scriven M 1972 Pros and cons about goal-free evaluation. Evaluation Comment 3 (4): 1–4

St. Augustine's lament cited in Rowntree D 1977 Assessing students How shall we know them? Harper and Row, London

Stalnaker J M 1951 The essay type of examination. In: Lindquist E F Educational measurement. George Banta Publishing, Menasha, Wisconsin

Stanley J C, Hopkins K D 1972 Educational and psychological measurement and evaluation, 5th edn. Prentice-Hall, Englewood Cliffs, N. J

Suchman E A 1977 Evaluating educational programs. In: Caro F G (ed) Readings in evaluation research. Russell Sage Foundation, New York

Taba H 1962 Curriculum development: theory and practice. Harcourt, Brace and World, New York

Thompson S 1979 A question of choice. Nursing Mirror 75 (30): 27–29

Thorndike R L, Hagen E 1977 Measurement and evaluation in psychology and education 4th edn. Wiley, New York

Tibbitts C E, Nicholas J R, McKay R J 1978 Unpublished paper — synopsis of which was published as Five teaching methods: a comparative study in nurse education. The Australian Journal of Education 22 (1): 91–92

Tyler R W 1942 General statement on evaluation. Journal of Educational research XXXV: 492–501

Vernon P E 1940 The measurement of abilities. University of London Press Ltd., London

Weiss C H 1972 Evaluation research. Prentice-Hall, N. J

Wiseman S 1949 The marking of English composition in grammar school selection. The British Journal of Educational Psychology XIX: 200–209

Chapter 5

Bloom B S (ed) 1956 Taxonomy of educational objectives Book 1 Cognitive domain. Longman, London

Boydell T 1976 Experiential learning. Department of Adult Education, University of Manchester

Campbell D T, Stanley J C 1966 Experimental and quasi-experimental designs for research. Rand McNally, Chicago

Entwistle N J 1973 The nature of educational research. (Block 1 of Educational studies: a third level course, methods of educational enquiry). Open University Press, Bletchley

General Nursing Council for Scotland 1973 Syllabuses for nursing (Reprint). General Nursing Council for Scotland, Edinburgh

Goodwin W L, Klausmeier H J 1975 Facilitating student learning. Harper and Row, New York

Gribble H E 1977 Gastro-enterological nursing. Nurses Aids Series, Special Interest Text. Balliere Tindall, London ·

Harrison J, Saunders M E, Sims A 1977 Integrating theory and practice in modular schemes for basic nurse education. Journal of Advanced Nursing 2 (5): 503–519

Information Services Division 1978 Scottish health statistics. HMSO, Edinburgh

Mager R F 1962 Preparing instructional objectives. Fearon Publishers, Belmont, California

Parlett M, Hamilton D 1972 Evaluation as illumination: a new approach to the study of innovatory programmes. Occasional Paper 9, Centre for Research in the Educational Sciences, University of Edinburgh

Tuckman B W 1978 Conducting educational research 2nd edn. Harcourt, Brace, Jovanovich, New York

Wilson S 1977 The use of ethnographic techniques in educational research. Review of Educational Research 47 (1): 245–265

Chapter 6

Burroughs G E R 1975 Design and analysis in educational research, 2nd edn.

Educational Monograph No. 8, University of Birmingham
Campbell D T, Stanley J C 1966 Experimental and quasi-experimental designs for research. Rand McNally, Chicago.
DHSS 1977 Directory of schools of nursing, 3rd edn. HMSO, London
General Nursing Council for Scotland 1978 Annual Report. General Nursing Council for Scotland, Edinburgh
Nie N H, Hull C H, Jenkins J G, Steinbrenner K, Bew D H 1975 SPSS — statistical package for the social sciences, 2nd edn. McGraw Hill, New York
Nie N H, Hull C H 1977 SPSS batch release 7.0 update manual. Programme Library Unit, University of Edinburgh
Pilliner A E G 1973 Experiment in educational research. (Block 5 of Educational studies: a third level course, methods of educational enquiry). Open University Press, Bletchley
Roethlisberger F J, Dickson W J 1939 Management and the worker. Harvard University Press, Cambridge, Massachusets
Siegel S 1956 Nonparametric statistics for the behavioral sciences. McGraw Hill, New York
Tuckman B W 1978 Conducting educational research, 2nd edn. Harcourt, Brace, Jovanovich, New York
Wright B D, Mead R J 1977 Bical: calibrating items and scales with the Rasch model. Research Memorandum No.23, Department of Education, University of Chicago

Chapter 7

DHSS 1977 Directory of schools of nursing, 3rd edn. HMSO, London
Hale S L 1974 An investigation of patient satisfaction and psycho-social aspects of nursing care. Unpublished PhD thesis, University of Maryland
Shields D 1978 Nursing care in labour and patient satisfaction: a descriptive study. Journal of Advanced Nursing 3 (6): 535–550

Chapter 9

Siegel S 1956 Nonparametric statistics for the behavioral sciences. McGraw Hill, New York

Chapter 10

Nuffield Provincial Hospitals Trust 1953 Work of nurses in hospital wards. Report of a job analysis. Nuffield Provincial Hospitals Trust, London

Chapter 12

Rogers C 1969 Freedom to learn. C E Merrill, Columbus, Ohio
Tuckman B W 1978 Conducting educational research, 2nd edn. Harcourt, Brace, Jovanovich, New York

Chapter 14

Wright B D, Mead R J 1977 Bical: calibrating items and scales with the Rasch model. Research memorandum No. 23, Department of Education, University of Chicago.

Chapter 17

Campbell D T, Stanley J C 1966 Experimental and quasi-experimental designs for research. Rand McNally, Chicago
Nuffield Provincial Hospitals Trust 1953 Work of nurses in hospital wards. Report of a job analysis. Nuffield Provincial Hospitals Trust, London

Chapter 18

Altschul A T 1980 Hints on maintaining patient-nurse interaction. Nursing Times 76 (15): 650–652

Bendall E 1975 So you passed, nurse. Royal College of Nursing and National Council of Nurses of the U.K., London

Birch J A 1972 An investigation into the cause of wastage during nurse training. Unpublished MEd thesis, University of Newcastle-upon-Tyne

Fretwell J E 1978 Socialisation of nurses: teaching and learning in hospital wards. Unpublished PhD thesis, University of Warwick

Gagné R M 1971 Instruction based on research in learning. Engineering Education 61: 519–523

General Nursing Council for Scotland 1976 Annual report. General Nursing Council for Scotland, Edinburgh

General Nursing Council for Scotland 1978 Annual report. General Nursing Council for Scotland, Edinburgh

General Nursing Council for Scotland 1980 Annual report. General Nursing Council for Scotland, Edinburgh

HMSO 1972 Report of the committee on nursing (The Briggs report). Cmnd 5115, HMSO, London

Hunt J M 1974 The teaching and practice of surgical dressings in three hospitals. Royal College of Nursing, London

Jones D C 1975 Food for thought. Royal College of Nursing, London

McGaghie W C, Miller G E, Sajid A W, Telder T V 1978 Competency-based curriculum development in medical education. (Public Health Papers No. 68) World Health Organisation, Geneva.

Marton F, Säljö R 1976 On qualitative differences in learning: I outcome and process. The British Journal of Educational Psychology 46 (Part 1): 4–11

Marton F, Säljö R 1976a On qualitative differences in learning: II Outcome as a function of the learner's conception of the task. The British Journal of Educational Psychology 46 (Part 2): 115–127

Ogier M E 1980 A study of the ward sister's leadership style and verbal interaction with nurse learners. Unpublished PhD thesis, University of London

Orton H D 1980 Ward learning climate and student nurse response. Unpublished MPhil thesis, Sheffield City Polytechnic

Pask G 1976 Styles and strategies of learning. British Journal of Educational Psychology 46 (Part 2): 128–148

Perry W G Jr. 1975 Intellectual and ethical development in the college years. In: Entwistle N J, Hounsell D J (eds) How students learn. Institute for Research and Development in Post-compulsory Education, University of Lancaster

Rogers C 1969 Freedom to learn. C E Merrill Publishing, Columbus, Ohio

Wong J 1979 The inability to transfer classroom learning to clinical nursing practice: a learning problem and its remedial plan. Journal of Advanced Nursing 4 (2): 161–168

World Health Organisation 1966 Expert committee on nursing: fifth report. Technical Report Series No. 347 World Health Organisation, Geneva

Further reading

This list has been selected from the bibliography of the original thesis. However, only references to material dated 1975 or later have been included here, and there are no references to theses, as these are not readily available to most readers. This list is in addition to the references.

Abdellah F G, Levine E 1979 Better patient care through nursing research, 2nd edn. Macmillan, London

Allen H O, Murrell J (eds) 1978 Nurse training. Macdonald & Evans, Plymouth

Barrows H S, Mitchell D L M 1975 An innovative course in undergraduate neuroscience experiment in problem based learning with 'problem boxes'. British Journal of Medical Education 9: 223–230

Boreham N C 1977 The use of case histories to assess nurses' ability to solve clinical problems. Journal of Advanced Nursing 2 (1): 57–66

Bruner J S 1975 Beyond the information given. In: Entwistle N J, Hounsell D J (eds) How students learn. Institute for Research and Development in Post-compulsory Education, University of Lancaster

Caro F G (ed) 1977 Readings in evaluation research, 2nd edn. Russell Sage Foundation, New York

Chater S 1975 Understanding research in nursing. World Health Organisation, Geneva

Clarke M 1977 Research in nurse education. Nursing Times Occasional Paper 73 (7): 25–28

Collins H W, Johansen J H, Johnson J A 1976 Educational measurement and evaluation, 2nd edn. Scott, Foresman, Glenview, Illinois

Combes R B 1977 Educating the learner to work on the ward. Nursing Times 73 (2): 46–47

Cullinan J 1979 The approach to post-basic teaching. Nursing Times 75 (17): 693

Dietrich G 1978 Teaching psychiatric nursing in the classroom. Journal of Advanced Nursing 3 (6) 525–534

Edmonds G, Musson V, Dixon E 1979 The specialist nurse teacher. Nursing Times 75 (37): 1586–1587

Ellis L, Podurgeil M, Palmer C 1979 Implementing a conceptual framework. Nursing Outlook 27 (2) 127–130

Entwistle N 1977 Changing approaches to research into personality and learning. Institute of Education. University of Göteborg

Erickson B H, Nosanchuk T A 1977 Understanding data. McGraw Hill, Ryerson, Toronto

Esther C A A, Bryant R J 1977 Educating learner to work on ward. Nursing Times 73 (2): 46–47

Fox D J 1976 Fundamentals of research in nursing, 3rd edn. Appleton Century Crofts, New York

Greaves F 1979 Teaching nurses in clinical settings I and II. Nursing Mirror Supplements 148 (8) and (9)

Haber A, Runyon R P 1977 General statistics. Addison-Wesley Publishing, London

Hall D C 1980 The nature of nursing and the education of the nurse. Journal of Advanced Nursing 5 (2): 149–159

Hamilton D 1976 Curriculum evaluation. Open Books, London

Hayter J 1979 How good is the lecture as a teaching method? Nursing Outlook 27 (4): 274–277

Hinchliff S M (ed) 1979 Teaching clinical nursing. Churchill Livingstone, Edinburgh

Huckabay L M 1978 Cognitive and affective consequences of formative evaluation in graduate nursing students. Nursing Research 27 (3) 190–194

Ianni F A J (ed) 1975 Conflict and change in education. Scott, Foresman, Glenview, Illinois

Infanté M 1975 The clinical laboratory in nursing education. Wiley, New York

Kilty M J 1976 Can nursing research learn from educational research? International Journal of Nursing Studies, 13: 97–102

Little D E, Carnevali D L 1976 Nursing care planning. Lippincott, Philadelphia

Mallick M J 1977 Do nursing educators preach what they want practised? Nursing Outlook 25(4): 244–247

Marson S N 1979 Nursing, a helping relationship? Nursing Times 29 (3): 541–544

Miller A E 1979 Nurses' attitudes towards their patients. Nursing Times 75 (45) 1929–1933

Moser C A, Kalton G 1977 Survey methods in social investigation, 2nd edn. Heinemann Educational, London

Perry S E 1979 Teaching strategy and learner performance. Journal of Nurse Education 18 (1): 25–27

Popham W J 1975 Educational evaluation. Prentice Hall, Englewood Cliffs, N. J.

Reid W A, Walker D F (eds) 1975 Case studies in curriculum change. Routledge and Kegan Paul, London

Revans R W 1978 The ABC of action learning. R W Revans, Publishers, Altrincham, Manchester

Rogers J (ed) 1978 Adults in education. BBC Publication, London

Ross M 1979 Accountability for nursing care — towards a new structure. Nursing Times 75 (27): 1478–1480

Royal College of Nursing of the United Kingdom 1976 New horizons in clinical nursing. Royal College of Nursing, London

Royal College of Nursing of the United Kingdom 1977 Ethics related to research in nursing. Royal College of Nursing, London

Schneider H L 1979 Evaluation of nursing competence. Little, Brown, Boston

Sheahan J 1978 Educating teachers of nursing: the contribution of educational studies. Journal of Advanced Nursing 3 (5): 447–455

Sheahan J 1978 Educating teachers of nursing: the contribution of pedagogical studies. Journal of Advanced Nursing, 3 (6): 515–524

Sheahan J 1979 Measurement in nursing education. Journal of Advanced Nursing 4 (1): 47–56

Sheahan J 1980 Educating teachers of nursing: a survey of the opinions of students. Journal of Advanced Nursing 5 (1) 71–81

Sims A 1976 Teachers of nursing in the United Kingdom and some characteristics of teachers and their jobs. Journal of Advanced Nursing 1 (5): 377–389

Spencer M 1979 Did the student learn? Nursing Times 75 (1): 35–37

Stenhouse L 1975 An introduction to curriculum research and development. Heinnemann, London

Tawney D (ed) 1976 Curriculum evaluation today: trends and implications. Macmillan Education, London

Thomas M C 1979 Study difficulties in undergraduate nursing students–a British perspective. International Journal of Nursing Studies 16 (4): 299–305

Tuckman B W 1975 Measuring educational outcomes: fundamentals of testing. Harcourt, Brace, Jovanovich, New York

Verhonick P J (ed) 1975 Nursing Research I. Little, Brown, Boston

Warcaba B 1976 An experimental scheme in nurse education. Journal of Advanced Nursing 1 (3): 243–252

Williamson J A (ed) 1976 Current perspectives in nursing education: the changing scene. Vol.I. Mosby, St Louis

Williamson J A (ed) 1978 Current perspectives in nursing education: the changing scene. Vol.II. Mosby, St Louis

World Health Organisation 1977 Report of the technical advisory group on the education of nursing/midwifery personnel. WHO, Copenhagen.

World Health Organisation 1977 Medium term programme in nursing/midwifery in Europe. WHO, Munich

Wright B D 1977 Solving measurement problems with the Rasch model. Journal of Educational Measurement 14 (2): 97–116

Appendix A

Care of patients with gastrointestinal conditions
Medical/surgical nursing

LEARNING OBJECTIVES — COGNITIVE

At the end of the course in the care of adult patients with disorders of the gastrointestinal system, the student nurse will be able to:

1. List and define common disorders/diseases.
2. Recall normal structure and function, and state how this is altered by disease.
3. Describe how the abnormal state will affect the patient, i.e. give the signs and symptoms.
4. Make relevant observations of the patient, and record and report these using appropriate terminology.
5. Name the investigative procedures used, explain the purpose of each, and list the nursing responsibilities in the preparation and care of the patient.
6. Define the various surgical operations.
7. Apply the relevant principles of nursing in planning and carrying out the care of individual patients with either a medical or surgical condition.
8. Assess priorities for nursing care in relation to individual patient's needs, at different stages in their illness.
9. Give reasons for each component of nursing care considered necessary for patients.
10. Name specific technical nursing procedures used in the care of such patients, and describe the nursing responsibilities involved in carrying out these procedures.
11. Evaluate the effects of nursing care given to individual patients.
12. Name possible complications, recognize the appropriate warning signs, and where relevant, state how such complications may be prevented or dealt with.
13. Relate theory to practice in all aspects of the nursing care of patients with disorders of the gastrointestinal system.

LEARNING OBJECTIVES — AFFECTIVE

At the end of the experimental course, it is hoped that the student nurse will:

A. Be aware of the different methods of providing patient care in terms of organisation by task assignment and patient assignment.

B. Be aware of, and value, the concept (idea) of individualised patient care, i.e. the provision of nursing care according to the individual needs of the particular patient, whatever method of organisation is current in the ward in which she is working at the time.

C. Incorporate the concept of individualised patient care into her own system of values, so that it becomes characteristic of her way of nursing.

Appendix B

Figures and Tables referred to in Chapter 14

(Presented in order as in that chapter)

Table B1 Tests and essays: sample of students for Part (1)

| College | Multiple choice test | | | | | | Essay test | | | |
| | Pre-test | | Post-test | | Retention test | | Post-essay | | Retention essay | |
	C	E	C	E	C	E	C	E	C	E
I	12	12	11	12	10	12	11	12	10	12
II	4	4	4	4	4	4	4	4	3	4
IV	8	8	8	8	8	7	8	8	8	7
V	8	8	8	8	8	8	8	8	8	8
Total N =	32	32	31	32	30	31	31	32	29	31

Note: C = control group students
E = experimental group students

College III students were omitted from the Table as there was no control group to contribute test scores in this college. There were however ten students in the experimental group who undertook all three multiple choice tests and their scores were analysed within their own college only. This separate analysis was also appropriate as these students were the 'one-off' group of more senior students.

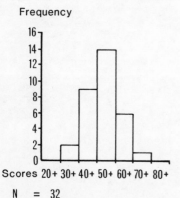

EXPERIMENTAL

Frequency

N = 32
M = 52·53
SD = 8·6
SE = 1·52

CONTROL

Frequency

N = 32
M = 52·63
SD = 9·16
SE = 1·62

Fig. B1 Histogram of pre-test scores: matched pairs

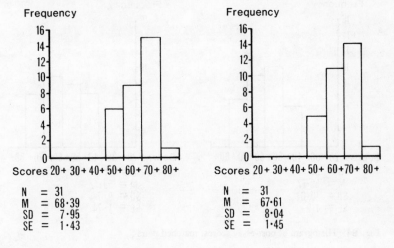

EXPERIMENTAL CONTROL

Fig. B2 Histogram of post-test scores: matched pairs

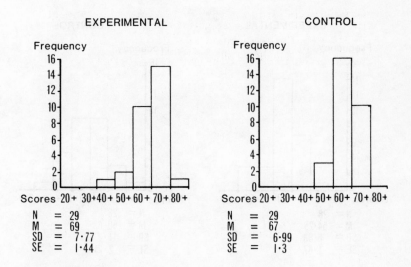

EXPERIMENTAL CONTROL

Fig. B3 Histogram of retention test scores: matched pairs

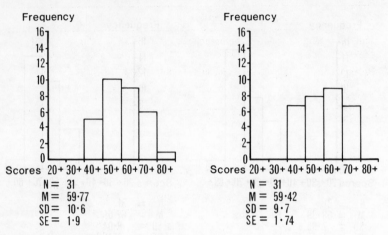

Fig. B4   Histogram of post-essay scores: matched pairs

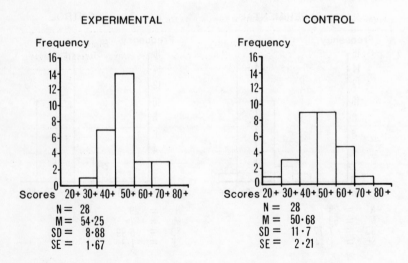

Fig. B5   Histogram of retention essay scores: matched pairs

Table B2 Tests and essays (within groups) : Pearson product moment correlations

Tests	Groups	N	r	s
Post-test with	Experimental	32	0.70	0.001
Post-essay	Control	31	0.48	0.01
Retention test with	Experimental	31	0.48	0.01
Retention essay	Control	29	0.53	0.01

Table B3 Tests and essays: sign test, direction of differences within pairs

Tests	No. of pairs	Differences (E - C) Positive	Negative	z	One-tailed probability
Post-test	31	16	15	0.000	NS
Post-essay	31★	16	14	0.183	NS
Retention test	29	19	10	1.486	0.07 (NS)
Retention essay	28	17	11	0.945	0.17 (NS)

★ = one 'tied' pair

Tables B4–B7 are on pages 244–247.

Table B8 Tests and essays: sample of students for Part (2)

College	Multiple choice test Pre-test	Post-test	Retention test	Essay test Post-essay	Retention essay
I	26	26	25	26	25
II	10	10	10	10	9
IV	24	24	22	24	22
V	21	21	20	21	20
Total N =	81	81	77	81	76

Table B4 Tests and essays: T-test, gain scores within groups

Tests	Group	N=	Mean	Standard deviation	Standard error	Difference between means	Standard error	T value	DF	1-tailed Probablity
Post-test to pre-test	Experimental	32	68.5625 52.5312	7.886 8.602	1.394 1.521	16.0312	1.327	12.08	31	<.001
Post-test to Pre-test	Control	31	67.6129 52.8064	8.049 9.257	1.446 1.663	14.8065	1.411	10.50	30	<.001
Retention test to Pre-test	Experimental	31	68.9032 52.1935	7.604 8.526	1.366 1.531	16.7097	1.148	14.55	30	<.001
Retention test to Pre-test	Control	30	67.3333 52.8333	7.107 9.414	1.298 1.719	14.5	1.37	10.58	29	<.001

Table B5 Tests and essays: T-test, loss scores within groups

Tests and essays	Group	N=	Mean	Standard deviation	Standard error	Difference between means	Standard error	T value	DF	1-tailed Probability
Retention test to Post-test	Experimental	31	68.9032	7.604	1.366	0.4516	1.044	0.43	30	NS
			68.4516	7.991	1.435					
Retention test to Post-test	Control	30	67.3333	7.107	1.298	−0.4333	1.327	−0.33	29	NS
			67.7667	8.14	1.486					
Retention essay to Post-essay	Experimental	31	54.5484	8.594	1.544	−5.0	1.497	−3.34	30	<.001
			59.5484	10.427	1.873					
Retention essay to Post-essay	Control	29	50.2758	11.692	2.171	−9.2069	1.870	−4.92	28	<.001
			59.4828	9.984	1.854					

Table B6 Tests and essays: T-test, difference scores within pairs

Tests and essays	Randomized blocks	No. of blocks	Mean difference	Standard deviation	Standard error	Difference between mean differences	Standard error of difference	T value	DF	2-tailed Probability
Pre-test to Post-test	Experimental	31	15.7419	7.447	1.338	0.9355	1.618	0.58	30	NS
	Control		14.8065	7.855	1.411					
Pre-test to retention test	Experimental	29	16.6207	6.472	1.202	2.1379	1.605	1.33	28	NS
	Control		14.4828	7.637	1.418					
Post-test to retention test	Experimental	29	0.8966	5.646	1.049	1.4138	1.833	0.77	28	NS
	Control		−0.5172	7.381	1.371					
Post-essay to retention essay	Experimental	28	−4.8929	8.293	1.567	3.3929	2.443	1.39	27	NS
	Control		−8.2857	8.923	1.686					

Table B7 Tests and essays: T-test, difference scores within groups, controlling for intervening practical experience

Tests and essays	Intervening experience	Group	N	Mean difference	Standard deviation	Standard error	T value	DF	2-tailed Probability
Post to retention test	Relevant	Experimental	21	1.4762	5.785	1.262	1.45	29	NS
	Not relevant		10	-1.7	5.539	1.752			
Post to retention test	Relevant	Control	15	0.6667	5.778	1.492	0.82	28	NS
	Not relevant		15	-1.5333	8.568	2.212			
Post to retention essay	Relevant	Experimental	21	-3.8571	8.645	1.886	1.11	29	NS
	Not relevant		10	-7.4000	7.486	2.367			
Post to retention essay	Relevant	Control	15	-6.8000	8.687	2.243	1.35	27	NS
	Not relevant		14	-11.7857	11.102	2.967			

Table B9   Tests and essays: means and standard deviations across and within colleges

Colleges	Essay average of 3 markers				Multiple choice test					
	Post- M (SD)	N	Retention M (SD)	N	Pre- M (SD)	N	Post- M (SD)	N	Retention M (SD)	N
All	60.00 (10.38)	81	56.36 (10.63)	76	53.7 (9.88)	81	68.52 (8.32)	81	68.48 (7.86)	77
I	59.87 (8.15)	26	51.32 (8.25)	25	53.12 (9.05)	26	70.04 (7.14)	26	69.00 (8.12)	25
II	58.47 (6.47)	10	54.67 (10.31)	9	52.7 (10.64)	10	71.90 (8.5)	10	69.5 (7.14)	10
IV	69.78 (6.27)	24	58.36 (11.48)	22	58.13 (10.33)	24	71.58 (7.38)	24	71.27 (8.3)	22
V	49.7 (7.5)	21	46.0 (9.0)	20	49.86 (8.60)	21	61.52 (6.85)	21	64.25 (5.86)	20

No essay from College III

Table B10   Tests and essays: Pearson product moment correlations, across and within colleges

College	Post-test with Post-essay			Retention test with Retention essay		
	N	r	s	N	r	s
All	81	0.60	0.001	76	0.53	0.001
I	26	0.43	0.01	25	0.16	N.S
II	10	0.65	N.S	9	0.72	0.01
IV	24	0.50	0.01	22	0.56	0.01
V	21	0.46	0.01	20	0.58	0.01

Table B11   Tests and essays: neutral marker means, standard deviations and range

Essays	N	Marker B			Marker C			Marker D		
		Mean	SD	Range	Mean	SD	Range	Mean	SD	Range
Post-essay	81	65.01	14.50	92–28	58.35	8.83	80–38	56.63	11.48	84–33
Retention essay	76	54.99	13.42	84–18	53.66	8.32	69–26	48.30	13.15	76–18

Table B12 Tests and essays: analysis of variance, post-essay

Source of variation	SS	DF	Mean square	F	Probability
Between subjects	25845.66255	80	323.07078		
Within subjects	10951.33333	162	67.60082		
Between judges	3176.79835	2	1588.39918	32.68927	<0.001
Residual	7774.53498	160	48.59084		
Total	36796.99588	242	152.05370		

Grand mean = 59.99588

Table B13 Tests and essays: analysis of variance, retention of learning essay

Source of variation	SS	DF	Mean square	F	Probability
Between subjects	25441.92982	75	339.22573		
Within subjects	8137.33333	152	53.53509		
Between judges	1903.13158	2	951.56579	22.89545	<0.001
Residual	6234.20175	150	41.56135		
Total	33579.26316	227	147.92627		

Grand mean = 52.31579

Table B14 Tests and essays: variation in neutral marker scores awarded to individual students

Essays	No. of students	Variation (in marks)		Mean
		Maximum	Minimum	
Post-essay	81	33	1	13.5
Retention essay	76	34	1	11.3

Table B 15 Tests and essays: neutral marker agreement as to pass or fail categorisation of students

Category	Post-essay		Retention essay	
	N	%	N	%
Agree to pass	54	67	34	45
Agree to fail	5	6	15	20
Disagree, but student passes	11	13.5	11	14
Disagree, but student fails	11	13.5	16	21
	81	100%	76	100%

Table B16   Tests and essays: Categorisation of students as pass or fail by individual markers

Markers	Post-essay Pass N	%	Fail N	%	Total N = 100%	Retention essay Pass N	%	Fail N	%	Total N = 100%
Marker B	70	86	11	14	81	46	61	30	39	76
Marker C	72	89	9	11	81	57	75	19	25	76
Marker D	57	70	24	30	81	38	50	38	50	76

Table B17   Tests and essays: T-test, difference scores within groups, controlling for intervening practical experience

Essays	N	Marker B with Marker C r	Marker B with Marker D r	Marker C with Marker D r
Post-essay	81	0.76	0.66	0.64
Retention essay	76	0.83	0.71	0.73

Index

Aim, of the experiment, 3, 75–76, 77,
   203
Apprenticeship
   and ward teaching, 140
   departures from the norm in the
     experiment, 203–204
   development *see* Nurse education and
     training
   model of training, 9, 11, 24, 73, 205

Bendall, E., 23, 27, 33, 39, 67, 215
Block system, 5, 15, 23, 217
   faults, 27
   inclusion of study periods, 192, 193
   timetable organisation, 92–93, 217
     insertion of the experiment, 93,
      96–98, 181

Campbell, D. T., and Stanley, J. C., 81,
   83, 84, 85, 204
Clinical nurse specialist, 125
Clinical teachers *see* Teachers of nurses;
   Ward teaching
Colleges of nursing and midwifery, 4–5,
   11
   survey of, 81, 205
   see also Block system
Confidentiality, 103, 106–107, 109, 110,
   189
Curriculum
   covert and overt, 4, 33
   critical criteria for development, 68
   evaluation, 68
   student preferences, 49

Data analysis, 88–89

Education and training *see* Nurse
   education and training
Enrolled nurses *see* Ward teaching;
   Ward trained staff
Ethical issues, 8–9
   see also Patients, consent to participate
Evaluation, 52, 62–69, 205
   analogy with drug trials, 64, 65
   and educational research, 65–66,
     67
   and nursing research, 66–68
   formative and summative, 64, 66
   functions, 62
   goal and goal-free, 64–65
   illuminative, 62, 68, 77–81
     aims, 79
     applied in the experiment, 79–82,
      204–205
     characteristics, 62–63
     defined, 78
   intrinsic, 64
   macro- and micro-, 64
   of nursing programmes, 28–29, 67
     by objectives, 18, 63, 69, 76,
      172–177
   pay-off, 64
   process and product, 63, 66, 67
   see also Experiment in integrating
     theory and practice; Test scores
     analysis; Tests and examinations
Examinations *see* Tests and examinations
Experiential learning, 38–43,
   158–179, 204, 205, 211, 220,
   222
   a continuum of meaning, 38
   applied in nursing, 40–43
     building upon natural potential, 40
     resisted, 40–41
     significant, 39, 41–42
   applied to the experiment, 162–163,
     165–169
     foundation for the experiment, 40,
      159

Experiment in integrating theory and
    practice
aims, 3, 75–76, 77, 203
assumptions, 9
context and approach, 4–5, 73–82
control group students' views,
    180–183, 212
control group teachers' views, 178,
    180–183, 212
defined, 3, 75, 86–87, 203
departures from the norm in nurse
    education and training, 203–204
design, 79, 80–81, 83–94, 204–205
effects
    upon patients, 170–173, 211
    upon students' learning, 162–169,
        181–183, 210–211
    upon ward routine, 159–161, 210
ethical issues, 8–9
evaluation
    by test scores see Test scores
        analysis
    qualitative, 158–183, 197–200
foundation, in learning theory, 40, 41
implementation details see Process of
    implementation
limitations, 9–10, 85–86, 187, 205
objectives, 75–77, 172–177, 212
    learning, 238–239
subject matter of teaching/learning
    course, 73–75
timetabling details, 92–94, 96–98,
    113
see also Evaluation, illuminative;
    Integration of theory and practice
Experimental training schemes
Canada, Ryerson Polytechnical
    Institute, 67
Glasgow, 17–18, 67, 68
modular, 27–28
St George's Hospital, London, 67
teaching methods, 36
    Bolton's introductory course,
        28–29

Flexi-time, 204
Freedom to learn, 38
see also Experiential learning; Rogers,
    C.

Gagné, R. M., 36, 45, 48

General Nursing Councils
creation, 12–13
promotion of modular training
    schemes, 27
GNC (England and Wales)
    and examinations, 53, 61
    single grade of teacher, 27
GNC (Scotland)
    and examinations, 53, 54
    and formulation of objectives, 28
    apprenticeship programme, 73, 74
    evidence to Royal Commission, 25
    new schemes of training, 28
    syllabus, 4, 92, 184
    teacher ratios, 220, 221
    teacher role, 25, 126, 206, 217
Gestalt
    concept applied to the experiment, 77
    theories of learning see Learning,
        Gestalt theories

Hamilton, D., see Parlett, M
Hartog P., and Rhodes, E. C., 58–59
Hawthorne effect, 84, 181, 183, 205, 212
Hypotheses, non-use discussed, 81–82

Integration of theory and practice, 3, 18,
    24, 28–29, 136–139, 166–167,
    173–177, 203–205, 207, 211,
    212, 214, 220, 225
an individual matter, 3, 30
and thinking, 29–30
demands, 29–30
discrepancies, 22–24, 134–136,
    137–138, 206, 207, 215
problems, 5–8
responsibility for, 17, 136, 152, 207
suggestions for improvement,
    138–139, 207
see also Experiment in integrating
    theory and practice; Transfer of
    learning

Knowledge
    and approach to nursing care, 47
    conception as contextual and relative,
        47, 221–222
    see also Experiential learning; Perry,
        W. G.

Learners' approaches to learning, 48–50, 224
a curriculum experiment, 49
cue-seeking, 50
deep or surface-level processing, 49–50
global or step-by-step, 48–49
holist or serialist, 48–49
influence of examinations *see* Tests and examinations

Learning
active (by doing) 41, 180, 211, 214, 221, 223
and individual differences, 37–38, 42, 43, 49, 223
and motivation, 36–38
and self-actualisation, 43
and the influence of examinations *see* Tests and examinations
as life-long process, 48
autonomous, 42
cognitive field theories *see* Gestalt
control/explore continuum, 36
discovery, 44, 221
'from the neck up', 38, 39, 222
from work experience, 6, 15
Gestalt theories, 34–36, 46
how to learn, 42, 165, 167, 204, 211, 224
in relation to Maslow's hierarchy of needs, 37
meaningful, 39, 43–44, 49, 222
provision of sub-sumers and advance organisers, 44
resistance to forgetting, 44
of principles, 16, 45, 50
process and outcome, 49
programmed (knowledge of results), 36
reception, 43
related to time interval between theory and practice, 27
retro-active inhibition, 45
rote, 50
stimulus-response, 34–36, 46
styles and strategies *see* Learners' approaches to learning
theories and concepts applied in nurse education, 31–51
to nurse education or training?, 32–34
transfer *see* Transfer of learning
trial and error, 35
see also Experiential learning
Learning climate, 41, 42, 43, 224

Main study, 80, 81, 84, 96–115, 205
timespan, 110–112
Marking of essay scripts
analytical marking, 58–59, 189–190
by college teachers, 109, 189
by neutral markers, 88, 109, 110, 184, 189–190, 213
impression marking, 58–59, 189–190, 213
reliability issue, 58–59, 184, 189–190
use of teams of markers, 58, 88, 190
see also Test scores analysis; Tests and examinations
Maslow, A., 37, 38, 42, 170, 222
Matching
learners' learning styles and teaching methods, 48–49
of student nurses in control and experimental groups, 85–86, 187, 212–213
see also Learners' approaches to learning
Measurement *see* Tests and examinations

Nurse education and training
'blunting' process, 40
development and dilemmas of apprenticeship system, 11–30, 205
early days, 11–12
influential middle years, 12–16
1940s to 1960s, 16–19
1970s, 19–29
the way forward?, 29–30
dichotomies, 22–28
experimental programmes *see* Experimental training schemes
in Scotland, 4–5
irrelevance to patient care, 24, 25
modular programmes, 5, 20, 24, 28, 220
potential for integration, 5
theories and concepts of learning applied, 31–51
Nursing
standards of care, 41, 42, 134–136, 139
effect of the experiment, 170–171, 177, 199, 211
see also Patients

Objectives
and criterion-referenced tests and testing, 55, 56

Objectives (*cont'd*)
General Nursing Council
recommendations, 28
levels of specificity, 76–77
of the experiment, 75–76, 238–239
achievement of, 172–177, 212
presentation to teachers, 99
of the Glasgow experiment, 17–18
Outcome measures, 82, 84, 87–88,
204–205

Parlett, M., and Hamilton, D., 78, 79
Patients
confidentiality of information, 107
consent to participate in the
experiment, 8, 91, 106
evaluation of care received, 106–107
needs, 167, 170–173, 211, 214–215,
221
satisfaction scale, 107
selection for inclusion in the
experiment, 105
'use' of, 214–215
Perry, W. G., 47, 222
Pilot study, 80, 81, 84, 95–96, 106, 195,
205
Process of implementation of the
experiment
accommodation for researcher, 106
availability of practical experience for
experimental group students, 98
day to day organisation, 107–108
determining student/teacher numbers,
98
meetings
with hospital nursing staff,
101–102, 112
with student nurses, 102–104, 112
with teachers, 96–99, 112
post-experiment procedures,
108–109, 112
questionnaire completion,
108–109, 112
pre-experiment procedures, 96–106,
112
questionnaire completion, 103,
105–106, 112
procedures during experiment,
106–108
record keeping, 107–108
retention stage procedures, 109–110,
112
follow-up questionnaire
completion, 110, 112

selection of patients, 105
timetabling details, 96–98, 113
see also Experiment in integrating
theory and practice; Sample

Questionnaires *see* Process of
implementation of the
experiment

Randomisation, 84–85, 187
Rasch item analysis model, 88, 184
Ratios
teachers to learners, 26, 216, 220–221
in the experiment, 98
ward staff to learners, 122
Reality shock, 24, 40, 138
Reliability, 57–59
Replication, 84, 205, 224
Reports
Briggs, 19–22, 27, 68, 217
Goldmark, 13
Horder, 16
Lancet, 13
Nuffield, 16, 134, 206
Platt, 18, 19
Research
educational, changing emphasis,
65–66, 78, 81
in nursing, 15, 17–19, 22–24, 25–29,
39, 40, 41, 66–68, 215
Research method
alternative paradigm, 78–79, 81
ethnographic techniques, 78
illuminative *see* Evaluation
experimental, 81, 83–84
pretest-posttest control group
design, 81, 84–85, 204
traditional approach, 81
agriculture-botany paradigm, 78
Rhodes, E. C. *see* Hartog, P.
Rogers, C., 38, 39, 40, 41, 42, 159, 222
principles of learning, 39–40
see also Experiential learning;
Freedom to learn

Sample, 89–91
colleges, 90, 123
hospitals, 91, 122, 158–159
patients, 91

Sample (*cont'd*)
  student nurses, 89, 120, 158, 191, 197, 240, 243
  teachers, 90–91, 123–127, 159
  ward trained staff, 91, 120–122, 158–159
Scott Wright, M., 17–19, 67
Self-esteem and self-actualization needs, 37, 38, 170, 211, 214–215
Significance testing, 88
  see also Test scores analysis
Staff nurses *see* Ward teaching; Ward trained staff
Stanley, J. C. *see* Campbell, D. T.
Student nurses
  as apprentices, 6, 33
  consent to participate in the experiment, 104, 198
  curricular preferences, 49
  learning needs, 18, 203, 209, 219
  opinions
    in programme evaluation, 67–68
    of the experimental method of teaching/learning *see* Experiment in integrating theory and practice
  perceptions of frequency of ward teaching received, 18, 141–147, 207
  study *see* Study patterns of student nurses
  supernumerary, 17, 19, 75, 140, 161, 221
  the difficult instructional moment, 47–48
  views about supervision, 163–164, 210
Study patterns of student nurses, 88, 131, 191–196, 213, 222, 223
  availability of study time in Block, 192, 193
  Block days represented in diaries, 191
  diaries, 88, 108, 191
  methods, 195
  self-initiated study, 194
  use of available study periods, 192–193
  variation between individuals, 194
  weekend study, 194
    link to examinations, 194
Summerhill, 38, 38n

Task assignment, 16, 86, 170, 171–173, 198, 212
Teachers
  as facilitators, 37, 42–43, 222–223
  demands of role, 42, 222
  see also Maslow; Rogers
Teachers of nurses
  clinical teacher, 7, 17, 26–27
    deployment, 124–125
    responsibility for ward teaching, 150
    role of tutor *vis à vis* clinical teacher as ward teacher, 152–153, 203, 209
    role of ward sister and staff nurse *vis à vis* clinical teacher as ward teacher, 154–155, 209
    see also Ward teaching
  contact with ward trained staff, 128–130, 162, 206
  continuance of two grades, 26, 27, 151–152, 218, 225
  deployment, 123–127, 206
  divorce from wards, 7, 15, 24–26, 216–218
    implications, 219–220
    reasons for separation, 25–26, 151–152
  generic role, 21, 26, 206, 217–218
  identical roles of both grades, 28–29, 203, 210, 218
  job satisfaction during the experiment, 162
  role in the experiment, 87, 161–162, 203, 210, 223
Teaching of nursing
  areas of uncertainty, 33–34
  class discussions, participation by student nurses, 131–133, 173–174, 196
  evaluated, 66–67
  methods used in the experiment
    advantages, 166–167, 211
    disadvantages, 167–169, 211
    effect upon subsequent nursing, 198–200
    feasibility, 178–179, 212
    for the control group students, 114, 182, 184
    for the experimental group students, 99–101, 114, 184
    general effectiveness, 162–169
  mix essential, 49, 223
  'spoonfeeding', 222, 223
  student nurse preferences, 131–133, 140, 208
  the difficult instructional moment, 47–48
  unrelated to ward practice, 133, 134–138

Teaching of nursing (*cont'd*)
'a happy accident', 14
Test scores analysis, 184–190, 212–213,
240–252
effect of intervening practical
experience, 188–189
feedback of results, 110
relationship between objective
(multiple choice) tests and
essay-format tests, 184, 186,
189–190, 213, 248
variation in pass/fail scores, 190, 213,
251, 252
Tests and examinations, 52–61
as predictors of practice, 23
criterion-referenced, 54–56
influence upon learning, 50–51
influence upon study *see* Study
patterns of student nurses
influence upon teaching, 57
national (State Final) 53, 59, 61, 184,
189
norm-referenced, 54–56
objective/subjective controversy,
57–58, 59–61
origins, 53–54
standardised, 53–54
teach-back testing technique, 48
teacher-made, 54
Tests, essay format, used in the
experiment
marks and marking *see* Marking of
essay scripts
post-essay administration, 108–109
reason for inclusion, 189
retention essay administration, 110
Tests, objective, used in the experiment,
50, 53–54, 57–58, 184
item analysis and marking, 88, 184
posttest administration, 108–109
pretest
administration, 103
as limit to generalisation, 85–86
as threat to validity, 83
structure and validation, 81
use in matching, 85–86, 185, 187,
212–213
retention test administration, 110
Theory and practice
defined, 4
relationship, 133
sequencing, 27–28, 220
setting for the research, 73–74
see also Block system; Bendall;
Learning; Integration of theory
and practice
Tool construction, 80–81

Total patient care, 167, 168, 170–173,
197–198, 211, 212, 214–215
an early proposal, 16
Transfer of learning, 45–47, 222
see also Learning

Ward sisters *see* Ward teaching; Ward
teaching methods; Ward trained
staff
Ward teaching, 14–15, 16–17, 38,
128–130, 140–155, 206–209
contribution of different staff grades,
as seen by student nurses,
141–149, 207–208, 215–216
enrolled nurses, 140–149
other student nurses, 140–149,
207–208
staff nurses, 128, 140–149, 206,
207, 208
teachers, 128–130, 140–147, 149,
203, 207, 208, 209
ward sisters, 140–149, 206, 207,
208, 209
opinions of teachers, 140, 150–151,
153, 154
reasons why not teaching in wards,
151–152
opinions of ward trained staff, 140,
149–151, 152–153, 154
responsibility for 150–151, 208–209,
219–220
tutor role *vis à vis* clinical teacher,
152–153, 203, 209
ward sister and staff nurse role *vis à vis*
clinical teacher, 154–155, 209
'use' of patients, 214–215
Ward teaching method used in the
experiment
opinions of experimental group
student nurses, 162–174,
210–212
opinions of teachers, 161, 162, 164,
165, 169, 171, 174–177, 210–212
opinions of ward trained staff, 164,
166–167, 169, 171, 174–177,
210–212
Ward teaching methods in use by ward
trained staff
by example, 148–149
supervision and practical
demonstration, 141–144, 148,
207
teaching at report time, 148–149
ward tutorials, 140, 143–147, 148,
207

Ward trained staff
  contact with teachers, 25, 128–130, 204, 206
  influence on students' behaviour, 24
  knowledge of students' theoretical preparation, 122–123, 206

Validity, 57–59

external, 83
internal, 83, 185
Values, 8, 10, 38, 40, 68, 77, 172, 196
  conflicting, betwixt education and service, 24, 25, 40
Variables, 81
  control of, 83, 85, 205
  dependent, 82, 87
  independent, 82, 86–87